Geriatric Psychiatry

What Do I Do Now?

SERIES EDITOR

Marc E. Agronin

PUBLISHED AND FORTHCOMING TITLES:
Child and Adolescent Psychiatry by Robyn P. Thom
and Christopher J. McDougle
Geriatric Psychiatry by Marc E. Agronin
and Ipsit V. Vahia

Geriatric Psychiatry

Edited by

Marc E. Agronin, MD, DFAPA, DFAAGP
Senior Vice President for Behavioral Health, Miami Jewish Health
Chief Medical Officer, MIND Institute at Miami Jewish Health
Affiliate Associate Professor of Psychiatry and Neurology,
University of Miami Miller School of Medicine
Miami, FL

Ipsit V. Vahia, MD, DFAAGP
Assistant Professor of Psychiatry, Harvard Medical School
Director, Technology and Aging Lab, McLean Hospital
Associate Chief of Geriatric Psychiatry
Medical Director of the Institute for Technology in Psychiatry
McLean Hospital
Belmont, MA

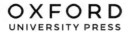

OXFORD
UNIVERSITY PRESS

OXFORD
UNIVERSITY PRESS

Oxford University Press is a department of the University of Oxford. It furthers
the University's objective of excellence in research, scholarship, and education
by publishing worldwide. Oxford is a registered trade mark of Oxford University
Press in the UK and certain other countries.

Published in the United States of America by Oxford University Press
198 Madison Avenue, New York, NY 10016, United States of America.

Library of Congress Cataloging-in-Publication Data
Names: Agronin, Marc E., editor. | Vahia, Ipsit V., editor.
Title: Geriatric psychiatry / [edited by] Marc E. Agronin, Ipsit V. Vahia.
Other titles: Geriatric psychiatry (Agronin) | What do I do now?. Psychiatry.
Description: New York, NY : Oxford University Press, [2022] |
Series: What do I do now? - psychiatry | Includes bibliographical references and index.
Identifiers: LCCN 2021058972 (print) | LCCN 2021058973 (ebook) |
ISBN 9780197521670 (paperback) | ISBN 9780197521694 (epub) |
ISBN 9780197521700 (online)
Subjects: MESH: Mental Disorders | Aged | Case Reports
Classification: LCC RC451.4.A5 (print) | LCC RC451.4.A5 (ebook) |
NLM WT 150 | DDC 618.97/689—dc23/eng/20220106
LC record available at https://lccn.loc.gov/2021058972
LC ebook record available at https://lccn.loc.gov/2021058973

DOI: 10.1093/med/9780197521670.001.0001

9 8 7 6 5 4 3 2 1

Printed by Marquis, Canada

To my wife Susie for her unwavering love, support and inspiration

Marc E. Agronin, MD

To my wife Stuti and my children Avik and Samik, who inspire me every day, and to my parents Vihang and Neela for their unconditional support.

Ipsit V. Vahia, MD

Contents

Preface xi

Contributors xiii

PART I ASSESSING THE GERIATRIC PATIENT

1 **What's happening to me?** 3
Cindy Marshall and Mary Quiceno

2 **Body, brain—and where the two meet** 15
Dustin Z. Nowaskie, Carol Chan, and Sophia Wang

3 **Mental status in the moment** 25
Zelde Espinel and Elizabeth A. Crocco

4 **Cognitive screens short and sweet—and when more is needed** 37
Kelly L. Konopacki and Sara L. Weisenbach

5 **A picture worth a thousand words** 45
Brandon Yarns and Aaron Greene

6 **What's normal and what's not? Putting it all together** 57
Saumil Dholakia, Sophiya Benjamin, and Joanne Ho

PART II NEUROCOGNITIVE DISORDERS

7 **Am I losing my mind?** 71
Angela M. Kristan and Elizabeth J. Santos

8 **I can't remember what just happened** 79
Michael Li and Erica C. Garcia-Pittman

9 **He became a different person practically overnight** 89
Matthew E. Kern, Jessica Stovall, and Prasad R. Padala

10 **The man who mistook the trash for his dog** 95
David Merril and Melita Petrossian

11 **Suddenly carefree and careless** 103
Anil Vatsavayi

12 **A telling triad of symptoms** 115
Fanny Huynh Du, Robert T. Hess, and Steve Huege

PART III ANXIETY DISORDERS

13 **I'm always afraid** 125
Maria Rueda-Lara and Elizabeth A. Crocco

14 **I felt as though I was about to die** 135
Rachel Zack Ishikawa and Feyza Marouf

15 **I can't get those thoughts out of my head** 145
Kalya Vardi

16 **Every reminder throws me off** 155
Azziza O. Bankole

PART IV MOOD DISORDERS

17 **To switch or to augment: That is the question** 167
Marie Anne Gebara and Jordan F. Karp

18 **Expecting the expected** 179
Susan W. Lehmann

19 **Life is not worth living** 185
Ali Asghar-Ali and Richa Lavingia

20 **Withering away** 195
Mario Fahed and Kristina Zdanys

21 **Sad or just unconcerned?** 203
Jennifer Junko Holiman, Kathryn Kieran, and Caroline S. Bader

PART V PSYCHOTIC DISORDERS

22 **It's like she lost her mind overnight** 211
Kripa Balaram, Deena J. Tampi, and Rajesh R. Tampi

23 **She thinks I'm someone else** 219
Silpa Balachandran, Deena J. Tampi, and Rajesh R. Tampi

24 **He is frightened of things that he sees** 227
Arshiya Syeda Farheen, Deena J. Tampi, and Rajesh R. Tampi

25 **Suspicious neighbors** 233
Michael Reinhardt, Muniza A. Majoka, and
Marco Christian Michael

26 **I live with these voices** 241
Tarek K. Rajji

PART VI OTHER DISORDERS

27 **Suddenly not the same** 249
Ipsit V. Vahia

28 **It's just a nightcap** 257
Luminita Luca and Elizabeth A. Crocco

29 **No one can work with her** 267
Marc E. Agronin

30 **Trustworthy or not?** 275
Karen Reimers

31 **Wired and ready** 283
Kathryn Kieran and Ipsit V. Vahia

Index 291

Preface

There is an instant paradox faced by any clinician working with older or geriatric patients. On the one hand, there are mostly the same psychiatric disorders that have the same basic symptomatic manifestations, require the same diagnostic steps, and respond to the same treatment modalities as with younger patients. It is important to keep these similarities in mind and not fall prey to stereotypes or ageist assumptions about older patients being necessarily more complex, impaired, and treatment resistant. Each person must be approached first and foremost like any other patient, and given the same amount of time, energy, and respect regardless of age. As obvious as this sounds, it is unfortunately true that many older patients are neglected by health systems that deem them too old and decrepit to be adequately diagnosed and treated.

On the other hand, each person regardless of age must be treated as a unique individual, and by this standard age *does* make a difference. There are unique age-conferred strengths of experience, knowledge, and wisdom that emerge during treatment and serve to humanize the patient and carry the day in therapeutic work. At the same time, there are age-conferred disorders and manifestations that are unique to many older patients and must be factored into clinical work. Chief among these differences is the role of neurocognitive impairment and disorders such as Alzheimer's disease that can profoundly influence diagnosis and treatment.

The purpose of this volume on geriatric psychiatry is to illuminate the commonalities and differences of the most common psychiatric diagnoses in older patients, and to provide clinicians with practical guides to answering the eponymous question when faced with clinical dilemmas: *What do I do now?*

Contributors

Marc E. Agronin, MD
Miami Jewish Health
MIND Institute at Miami Jewish
Health
Department of Psychiatry and
Neurology
University of Miami Miller School
of Medicine
Miami, FL, USA

Ali Asghar-Ali, MD
Menninger Department of
Psychiatry and Behavioral Sciences
Baylor College of Medicine
Houston, TX, USA

Caroline S. Bader, MD
Department of Geriatric Psychiatry
McLean Hospital
Belmont, MA, USA

Silpa Balachandran, MD
Cleveland Clinic Akron General
Akron, OH

Kripa Balaram, MD
Department of Psychiatry
MetroHealth Medical Center
Cleveland, OH, USA

Azziza O. Bankole, MD
Department of Psychiatry and
Behavioral Health
Virginia Tech Carilion School of
Medicine
Roanoke, VA, USA

Sophiya Benjamin, MBBS, FRCPC
Department of Psychiatry and
Behavioural Neurosciences
McMaster University
Hamilton, ON, CA

Carol Chan, MBBCH, MSc
Department of Psychiatry
Case Western Reserve University
School of Medicine
Cleveland, OH, USA

Elizabeth A. Crocco, MD
Department of Psychiatry and
Behavioral Sciences
University of Miami Miller School
of Medicine
Miami, FL, USA

**Saumil Dholakia, MBBS, MD,
MHSc (Bioethics)**
Department of Psychiatry
University of Ottawa
Ottawa, ON, CA

Fanny Huynh Du, MD
Division of Neuromuscular
Medicine
Department of Neurology and
Neurological Sciences
Stanford University
Stanford, CA, USA

Zelde Espinel, MD
Department of Psychiatry
University of Miami
Miami, FL, USA

Mario Fahed, MD
Department of Psychiatry
University of Connecticut
Health Center
Farmington, CT, USA

Arshiya Syeda Farheen, MD
Department of Psychiatry and
Psychology
Cleveland Clinic Akron General
Akron, OH, USA

**Erica C. Garcia-Pittman,
MD, FAPA, DFAAGP**
Associate Professor
Program Director, Geriatric
Psychiatry Fellowship
Psychiatry and Behavioral Sciences
Dell Medical School | The
University of Texas at Austin
Austin, TX, USA

Marie Anne Gebara, MD
Department of Psychiatry
University of Pittsburgh
Pittsburgh, PA, USA

Aaron Greene, MD
Department of Psychiatry and
Biobehavioral Sciences
David Geffen School of Medicine
at the University of California Los
Angeles
Los Angeles, CA, USA

Robert T. Hess, MD
Department of Neurosciences
University of California, San Diego
San Diego, CA, USA

Joanne Ho, MD, FRCPC, MSc
Department of Medicine, Division
of Geriatric Medicine, Division
of Clinical Pharmacology and
Toxicology, Division of Innovation
and Education
McMaster University
Kitchener, ON, CA

**Jennifer Junko Holiman, MSN,
APRN/CNP, PMHNP-BC**
Department of Geriatric Psychiatry
McLean Hospital
Belmont, MA, USA

Steve Huege, MD, MSEd
Department of Psychiatry
UCSD School of Medicine
La Jolla, CA, USA

**Rachel Zack Ishikawa,
PhD, MPH**
Department of Psychiatry
Massachusetts General Hospital
Boston, MA, USA

Jordan F. Karp, MD
Department of Psychiatry
University of Arizona
Tucson, AZ

Matthew E. Kern
Wake Forest School of Medicine

Kathryn Kieran, MSN, PMHNP-BC
Department of Geriatric Outpatient Psychiatric Clinic and Research Programs
McLean Hospital
Belmont, MA, USA

Kelly L. Konopacki, PhD
Department of Psychiatry
University of Utah
Salt Lake City, UT, USA

Angela M. Kristan, MD
Department of Psychiatry
Gianna of Syracuse Medical PLLC
Pittsford, NY, USA

Richa Lavingia, MD
University of Pittsburgh
Medical Center
Pittsburgh, PA, USA

Susan W. Lehmann, MD
Department of Psychiatry and Behavioral Sciences
The Johns Hopkins University School of Medicine
Baltimore, MD, USA

Michael Li, MD
Department of Psychiatry
The University of Texas Southwestern Medical Center
Dallas, TX, USA

Luminita Luca, MD, PhD
Department of Psychiatry and Behavioral Health
University of Miami
Miami Shores, FL, USA

Muniza A. Majoka, MBBS
Department of Psychiatry
Yale School of Medicine
New Haven, CT, USA

Feyza Marouf, MD
Boston Center for Memory
Boston, MA, USA

Cindy Marshall, MD
Department of Neurology
Baylor University Medical Center
Dallas, TX, USA

David Merril, MD, PhD
Pacific Brain Health Center
Pacific Neuroscience Institute
Santa Monica, CA, USA

Marco Christian Michael, MD
Department of Psychiatry and Behavioral Sciences
SUNY Downstate Health Sciences University
Brooklyn, NY, USA

Dustin Z. Nowaskie, MD
Department of Psychiatry
Indiana University School of Medicine
Indianapolis, IN, USA

Prasad R. Padala, MD
Department of Psychiatry
University of Arkansas for Medical
Sciences
Little Rock, AR, USA

Melita Petrossian, MD
Pacific Movement Disorders Center
Pacific Neuroscience Institute
Santa Monica, CA, USA

Mary Quiceno, MD
Internal Medicine & Geriatrics
University of North Texas Health
Science Center
Fort Worth, TX, USA

Tarek K. Rajji, MD, FRCPC
Toronto Dementia Research
Alliance
University of Toronto
Toronto, ON, CA

Karen Reimers, MD
Department of Psychiatrist
University of Minnesota, University
of Central Florida
Clearwater, FL, USA

Michael Reinhardt, MD
Department of Psychiatry
SUNY Downstate Health Sciences
University
Brooklyn, NY, USA

Maria Rueda-Lara, MD
Department of Psychiatry
University of Miami
Miami, FL, USA

Elizabeth J. Santos, MD, MPH
Departments of Psychiatry,
Neurology and Medicine
University of Rochester School of
Medicine and Dentistry
Rochester, NY, USA

Jessica Stovall
University of Arkansas for Medical
Sciences

Deena J. Tampi, MD
Behavioral Health Advisory Group
Princeton, NJ

**Rajesh R. Tampi, MD, MS,
DFAPA, DFAAGP**
Department of Psychiatry
Creighton University School of
Medicine
Omaha, OH, USA

Ipsit V. Vahia, MD
Department of Geriatric Psychiatry
McLean Hospital/Harvard
Medical School
Belmont, MA, USA

Kalya Vardi, MD
Division of Geriatric Psychiatry
University of California San Diego
La Jolla, CA, USA

Anil Vatsavayi, MD, MPH
Department of Psychiatry
Harvard Medical School
Boston, MA, USA

Sophia Wang, MD, MS
Department of Psychiatry
Indiana University School of
Medicine
Indianapolis, IN, USA

Sara L. Weisenbach, PhD
Department of Psychiatry &
Behavioral Health
Stony Brook University
Stony Brook, NY, USA

Brandon Yarns, MD, MS
Department of Mental Health
VA Greater Los Angeles
Healthcare System
Los Angeles, CA, USA

Kristina Zdanys, MD
Department of Psychiatry
University of Connecticut School
of Medicine
Farmington, CT, USA

PART I

Assessing the Geriatric Patient

1 What's happening to me?

Cindy Marshall and Mary Quiceno

A 65-year-old man presents with anxiety. He reports that for the last 6 months he has been repeatedly checking faucets to see if the water is turned off and going into the garage to make sure he turned off the light. He also describes mild cognitive changes including short-term memory lapses and word-finding difficulty when making sales presentations at work. As a result, his sales volume at work has declined, and he has been put on probation. His sister notes a change in his personal grooming and dress. He has greeted guests at his front door while wearing only his underwear. During the interview, he is noted to be picking at his fingers. He responds to questions asked of him but does not contribute information spontaneously.

What do you do now?

STARTING THE HISTORY-TAKING

Without a comprehensive history it's difficult if not impossible to formulate potential diagnoses. Participation of a collateral informant is ideal. If a person comes alone, ask for assent to call someone who knows them well and is familiar with their situation. Be sensitive to the fact that someone other than the patient may have scheduled the appointment. Individuals with memory disorders may assert they were never told about the visit and they may lack insight into the presenting problems. Even before you begin, then, the patient may be confused as to why they are seeing you, and filled with strong emotions such as fear, resentment, or anger.

THE ART OF COMMUNICATION

In order to learn the most from the patient and informant, it's important to establish rapport early on. Introduce yourself and state your role. Ask open-ended questions that require more than a "yes" or "no" answer. You may draw upon the patient's own background, knowledge, or feelings to get them talking. Even when the patient is resistant to the evaluation, a skillfully planned conversation will induce them to demonstrate key neurocognition abilities such as attention, orientation, memory, knowledge, and both receptive and expressive language. Be an attentive listener. Use "we" and "us" pronouns to convey a collaborate process between you and the patient and their informants. With older patients especially, it is crucial to not be rushed or dismissive. Always respond with respect and empathy for the individual's background, season of life, and desire for autonomy. Older adults have a wealth of life experiences that will provide ample opportunities for exploring their present situation through a discussion about their past history. Because many older adults may have challenges related to vision or hearing, clarify this and be prepared to change the tone and/or volume at which you speak to suit the patient's comfort level.

With the man in question, he was distractible during the interview and required redirection and engagement of his sister to keep him involved and on track. The interviewer remained patient and pleasant with him, and asked him about several of his interests to get him talking.

HISTORY OF PRESENT ILLNESS

Once you establish rapport through your initial greetings and conversation, you need to obtain a detailed history of the present illness (HPI). Ask the patient and then the informant the reason for the visit. Start with open-ended questions such as: What is going on? What brought you here? How can I help? Use their narrative to make observations regarding their ability to express themselves, provide an organized timeline, stay on track, and have insight into their problems. Categorical prompting can increase the amount of information elicited. Ask for specific examples of problem areas in cognition, functioning, and behavior as outlined in Table 1.1.

The questions you ask about mood, perception, and thought process and content will supplement and clarify the mental status examination (MSE). For example, someone who reports a history of hallucinations might not be demonstrating them during the appointment, or they might report a history of visual disturbances that indicate a specific nonpsychotic etiology. With all of these issues, history-taking, whether conducted before, during, or after the MSE, is a critical component to provide context.

Although the 65-year-old man and his sister had already provided a very detailed description of his current symptoms, the structured HPI filled in many other details, including more pronounced difficulty with communicating at work and organizing his sales data, other incidents of inappropriate behaviors such as making crude comments to family members and coworkers, and an increased focus on eating sugary breakfast cereals for many of his meals.

PAST MEDICAL HISTORY

The past medical history can cover many different conditions, so you might consider prompting the patient and informant with a written checklist to cue recall. Use any available paper and electronic medical records, but don't assume they are complete. Explore the medical history for comorbidities that contribute to neuropsychiatric presentations such as stroke, movement disorders, head injuries, sleep apnea, vitamin deficiencies, infection, and thyroid dysfunction.

The patient was in remarkable physical shape for his age, and a thorough review of recent medical records and labs did not reveal any potential causes for

TABLE 1.1 How the HPI can reveal cognitive and functional changes

To learn about	Ask about
Complex attention	Concentration; distractibility; multitasking
Learning and memory	Forgetfulness; repetitive questions; missed appointments
Language ability	Word-finding difficulty or word substitution; loss of word meaning; naming issues; trouble understanding instructions
Executive functioning	Problem-solving; decision-making; organization; judgment
Perceptual-motor abilities	Ability to use appliances and other items; following maps or directions to someplace
Social cognition	Disinhibition or other inappropriate behaviors; loss of empathy or insight
Activities of daily living	Feeding; dressing; toileting; bathing
Instrumental activities of daily living	Meal preparation; medical and financial preparation
Driving	Getting lost; accidents; unexplained scrapes on car; road rage
Occupational performance	Poor performance evaluations at work; unable to master new tasks; loss of job; or early retirement
Motor abilities/gait	Falls; rigidity; slowed movements; tremors
Mood	Presence, degree, and frequency of mood swings; depression; anxiety; euphoria; anger; irritability
Thinking	Distortions; disorganization; slowed or speeded up thinking
Thoughts	Delusions (e.g., paranoid ideas, misidentification); obsessions; suicidal thoughts; homicidal thoughts

TABLE 1.1 **Continued**

To learn about	Ask about
Perceptions	Presence, type, frequency, triggers, and reactions for hallucinations
Sleep	Ability to fall asleep and stay asleep; interruptions; early morning awakening; behaviors during sleep
Appetite	Increases; decreases; specific preferences
Substance use	Routine use of alcohol, cannabis, narcotics, and others

his neurocognitive and behavioral symptoms. He was only listed as having hyperlipidemia and benign prostatic hypertrophy.

MEDICATIONS AND ALLERGIES

Updated medication lists are essential but can be difficult to get, even when you have medical records. It's best to review any list with both patient and informant, and consider having them bring in all of their medication bottles if necessary. Ask the patient to specify dosing times due to potential impact on efficacy, tolerability, and function. Be mindful that any list might not represent exactly what the patient is actually taking, so ask about adherence. Sometimes you need blood levels (e.g., with lithium or Depakote) to confirm adequate dosing and adherence. Always inquire about over-the-counter medications and supplements, especially for sleeping pills. Ask about as-needed or PRN use and focus on medications that have significant side effects in the elderly, such as anticholinergics, benzodiazepines, muscle relaxants, and narcotics. The Beers List is an important resource to consult since it lists all of the medications that are risky to use in older individuals. Finally, obtain a list of all drug and food allergies, which should include any medications that were not tolerated due to various side effects.

The patient was taking a statin medication and denied anything else. However, his sister found dozens of bottles of various vitamins and supplements at his house, including several touted to help his prostate health.

By reviewing all of these pill bottles, she and the doctor realized that he was compulsively shopping on certain websites and buying large quantities of unnecessary pills. Several of them contained caffeine and other potentially stimulating herbal products.

PAST PSYCHIATRIC HISTORY

Inquire about past diagnoses and treatment for the major categories of psychopathology: mood disorders, anxiety disorders, psychotic disorders, substance use disorders, and neurocognitive disorders. It may be more difficult to get histories of personality disorders and somatoform disorders, so ask about recurrent conflicts with others and chronic physical complaints. With each disorder, inquire about common symptoms and manifestations and course, including depression, mania, suicide attempts, panic attacks, hallucinations, and various forms of delusional thinking. Investigate the history of treatment, including psychotherapy, medication trials and response, electroconvulsive therapy (ECT) and transmagnetic stimulation (TMS), and psychiatric hospitalizations (both intensive/partial outpatient and inpatient).

The patient had a previous history of mild anxiety following a divorce several decades prior and had had psychotherapy and a brief trial of a benzodiazepine. He also reported insomnia and revealed that he used an over-the-counter cough syrup to help him sleep, but none in the last 10 years.

FAMILY HISTORY

Family history may give a clue to the diagnosis, especially when there is either a first-degree relative with a specific disorder or multiple siblings or other relatives with it. Having a parent with a chronic psychotic disorder, suicidality, or substance use disorder may not only provide clues to the patient's diagnosis, but also raise the possibility of traumatic childhood experiences. Age of onset of the family member's symptoms could provide a clue to an autosomal dominant disorder, especially with Alzheimer's disease. Mood, anxiety, and substance use disorders often run in families, but remember that the onset of these symptoms much later in life may indicate weaker genetic roots.

The patient had a maternal aunt who suffered from an unspecified form of dementia in her 50s, with some symptoms that sounded similar to his current presentation. She died many years ago, however, and no one knew her exact diagnosis.

PREVIOUS ASSESSMENTS

Previous assessment are part of both past and current medical and psychiatric history and can aid in establishing the differential diagnosis and filling in gaps in your understanding of the etiology of the patient's symptoms. Some of the key assessments to obtain previous records for (or to include in your own evaluation) are:

- Physical and neurologic examinations
- Laboratory data
- Neuroimaging (CT, MRI, and PET scans)
- Sleep studies
- Electroencephalogram (EEG)
- Cerebrospinal fluid analysis
- Neuropsychological testing

Often, these studies will provide a baseline for comparison and a rule-out of certain factors, such as previous stroke or tumors, rather than a definitive diagnosis.

Our patient's annual physical exam and lab data were all normal. He had a previous MRI of his brain and an EEG in the last year, which both were normal. He also had a sleep study several years ago; it showed no sleep apnea or other abnormalities.

SOCIAL HISTORY

The social history will accomplish two primary goals of teaching you about your patient's background and current living situation. Often, these details can prompt friendly conversations that can open up the interview, keep it flowing, and help you bond with the patient and informant. When you learn about their background, try to find areas of commonality (e.g., you and the patient are avid sports fans) or interest (e.g., you are intrigued by the patient's artistic abilities) that you can ask about to establish rapport and foster a trusting and empathic relationship. These topic areas serve to humanize the person behind the patient or diagnosis. Several key areas to inquire about are:

- Origins (time, place, and circumstances of birth and childhood)
- Family of origin (parents, siblings, other significant figures)
- Religion, ethnicity, and nationality
- Educational background
- Occupation(s) and post-retirement roles
- Marriage and family (number, length, children, grandchildren, and other offspring)
- Major life events (e.g., historical experiences, trauma, life-changing illnesses or injuries, major losses, wartime experiences)
- Current living situation (location, type of residence, with whom)
- Current stresses (physical or mental disabilities, social needs, financial resources and challenges) and available in-home and other sources of assistance

These details are often relegated to a short paragraph at the end of many histories, or are not even included except for a few demographic details, and yet they are often some of the most important aspects of a person's life and will motivate the entire doctor–patient relationship. They will also reveal the many strengths the person has in addition to their problems and challenges.

A discussion with the patient revealed him to be a hugely successful salesperson with a larger-than-life personality and many hobbies, including fly fishing and boating. The interviewer loved fishing and was able to draw out the patient by talking about their mutual love, and this became a way for the patient to bond with the doctor and remember the appointments better and with positive feelings. It gave the doctor a sense of how much the patient's personality had changed over time, which was revealing of the existence of frontal lobe impairment. Ultimately, it would also provide ideas for how to keep the patient engaged in meaningful activities even as he would become unable to work or function independently.

REVIEW OF SYSTEMS AND FUNCTIONAL ASSESSMENT

Even though you will have a medical history, it is important to quiz the patient and informant about any current physical symptoms from head to toe, covering all major physiologic systems in the body. A checklist often helps in this regard. Current or recent symptoms revealed by the review of these systems, such as headaches, appetite changes, constipation, incontinence, and back pain, will help to understand the patient's daily life and the potential effects of other disorders and medications. It will also help round out the differential diagnosis. At the same time, it is important to translate all of the medical and cognitive issues into the practical or functional effects on the person's daily life, known as their activities of daily living (ADLs). The main ADLs include bathing/showering, personal hygiene/grooming, dressing, feeding oneself, using the bathroom, and ambulation. Higher-level *instrumental* ADLs include preparing meals, shopping, taking medications, managing money, using the telephone, cleaning up one's living space, and traveling outside the home. There are several scales that can be used to assess these easily and that can be incorporated into routine assessments.

The patient was having frequent headaches and loose stools. These symptoms appeared to be linked to two other details revealed in the patient's history: his use of multiple stimulating herbal supplements (causing headaches) and excessive consumption of sugary breakfast cereals (causing loose stools). When both of the factors were controlled, the symptoms revealed by the review of systems cleared up. His ADLs were generally intact, although he was beginning to show some neglect for his personal hygiene even though he appeared to know what to do. He was starting to have some minor trouble with several instrumental ADLs, including keeping his home clean, shopping, and managing his money appropriately, all further reflective of evolving frontal lobe changes.

CAREGIVER ISSUES

The care partner and other informal and professional caregivers are the key to obtaining history and implementing your diagnostic and therapeutic plans. It is critical to have permission to communicate with the most important caregivers and to have ways for them to reach you and provide updates and get questions answered. The basic information you will need to complete a caregiver profile includes:

- Who currently provides care?
- What are their schedules and availability?
- What sort of supervision and care is being provided? What is still needed?
- Is the current living situation safe?
- Are there any concerns about caregiver burnout, incompetence, abuse, or neglect?
- Is a higher level of care needed (e.g., assisted living, memory care, or nursing home)?

Keep in mind that the informants present at visits may be reluctant to share certain details due to fear of upsetting the patient or causing an argument. As a result, they may want to talk to you separately. An additional question that should always be included is how the primary caregiver is doing in terms of their own stress.

The patient has been living alone and has no caregiver other than his sister, who sees him several times a week. She is noticing increased problems with his personal hygiene, home cleanliness, and inappropriate behaviors, and feels that he needs help at home. She is extremely concerned and stressed about the situation.

NEEDING AN INTERPRETER

It is not unusual for clinicians to encounter patients for whom English is not their first language. If a patient is more comfortable communicating in a language other than English, clinicians are best served using interpreter services to communicate directly with the patient rather than relying on proxy information. Several hospitals and clinics provide interpreter services, and clinicians should use these. Services may include access to a person who participates in person and serves as an interpreter, phone-based services, or, more recently, app-based services. When working with an interpreter it is preferable to ask the interpreter to translate questions and responses verbatim rather than provide explanations, since this may introduce the interpreter's own biases into the discussion. While family members or caregivers may offer to serve as interpreters, this should be avoided.

PUTTING IT ALL TOGETHER

Once you complete the basic history, you need to ask yourself: Did I miss anything? Then ask the patient and informant: Is there an issue you wanted to mention that I didn't ask about? Because older adults commonly present with both psychiatric and neurocognitive symptoms, timelines are instrumental for organizing the history. The current presentation may be consistent with a new or recurrent psychiatric disorder, or it could be an emerging neurocognitive disorder.

In addition, all neurocognitive disorders have associated psychiatric symptoms, which are sometimes appreciated only in retrospect. For example, behavior changes, apathy, and obsessive-compulsive symptoms may be early manifestations of frontotemporal neurocognitive disorder. Alzheimer's disease may initially present with depression and apathy. Hallucinations may be a harbinger of neurocognitive disorder due to Lewy bodies. The timeline of change in the person's overall history will help to shape the differential diagnosis.

With this patient, the timeline clearly shows early onset of behavioral disinhibition and neurocognitive changes that are completely new for the patient, who had no previous psychiatric history. There are no clear medical or medication-related factors that would likely cause these changes. His MRI was unrevealing. As a result, a frontotemporal dementia is considered likely, and further diagnostic tests will be ordered.

KEY POINTS TO REMEMBER

- It is important to establish rapport with older patients and actively include informants and other caregivers in the history-taking.
- The basic history in older adults should include detailed questions about every area of neurocognition function.
- There is often a lot of past medical and psychiatric history and multiple medications for older patients, which requires mining both paper and electronic records to corroborate the reported history.

- The social history will help humanize the patient and provide information to build rapport as well as begin to assess the influence of the current social network.
- The review of systems provides perspective on current physical complaints and limitations and helps to assess current physical and sensory functioning.
- Caregiver history is critical to assessing the safety and integrity of the patient's current living situation, including the role and competence of the caregivers involved in daily life.

Further Reading

Fortin AH, Dwamena FC, Frankel RM, Lepisto BL, Smith RC. *Smith's Patient-Centered Interviewing: An Evidence-Based Method* (4th ed.). McGraw Hill; 2018.

Gerolimatos LA, Gregg JJ, Edelstein BA. Interviewing older adults. In: Pachana NA, Laidlaw K, eds. *Oxford Handbook of Clinical Geropsychology*. Oxford University Press; 2014:163–183.

History Taking: Overview. Oxford Medical Education. https://www.oxfordmedicaleducation.com/history/medical-general/

Woolley JD, Khan BK, Murthy NK, Miller BL, Rankin KP. The diagnostic challenge of psychiatric symptoms in neurodegenerative disease; rates of and risk factors for prior psychiatric diagnosis in patients with early neurodegenerative disease. *J Clin Psychiatry.* 2011;72(2):126–133.

2 Body, brain—and where the two meet

Dustin Z. Nowaskie, Carol Chan, and Sophia Wang

The patient is a 75-year-old man with a past history of depression, hypertension, type 2 diabetes mellitus, and hyperlipidemia. He has been referred to you by his primary care provider for "memory issues and cognitive decline." Over the past year the patient has noticed short-term memory changes, word-finding difficulties, and worsening depressive symptoms, including anhedonia and insomnia. He reports two falls with mild head injuries over the prior month, but no medical assessment. His partner has had to assume greater responsibility for cooking, cleaning, managing finances, and driving. You suspect that the patient has a progressive neurocognitive disorder and have to decide on what medical and neurologic tests to order.

What do you do now?

A complete medical and examination should be completed during the assessment for potential neurocognitive disorders. The standard medical exam follows complete history-taking, described in Chapter 1, and includes vital signs, physical and neurologic examination, and then more specific assessments and laboratory tests guided by the differential diagnosis.

VITALS AND PHYSICAL EXAM

A complete set of vital signs includes the pulse rate, blood pressure, respiration rate, oxygen saturation (via pulse oximetry), body temperature, and an assessment of pain. It is important to measure orthostatic pulse rate and blood pressure if orthostatic hypotension is suspected or if symptoms such as weakness, ambulation/balance difficulties, dizziness, and/or lightheadedness are endorsed. The elements of a complete physical exam relevant to the older psychiatry patient are listed in Table 2.1.

The extent of the medical exam depends on the chief complaint and the practice preferences of the examiner. While some clinicians perform a complete medical exam regardless of the etiology, generally most perform a focused exam based on the history and review of systems.

NEUROLOGIC ASSESSMENT

A thorough neurologic examination should be completed during the assessment for potential neurocognitive disorders (Table 2.2).

The decision to add more specific tests should be guided by the differential diagnosis. Any neurologic clues can be observed from the history-taking and conversation with the patient. For example, observation of the patient's speech, ability to recall recent events, and any abnormal movements may provide signs of neurologic deficits even before the formal neurologic exam has begun.

A standard assessment of the cranial nerves should be performed, with particular attention paid to areas that may be associated with cognitive impairment. For example, patients with Alzheimer's disease or other dementias such as Parkinson's disease dementia and Lewy bodies dementia may experience anosmia even early in the disease. In early stages of neurodegenerative dementias, abnormalities in extraocular movements are generally

TABLE 2.1 **Physical examination**

System	Pertinent findings
Constitutional	Distress level, psychomotor agitation or retardation, overall appearance
HEENT	Appearance of the head, eyes/sclera, ears, and mucous membranes; movement of the extraocular muscles; visual and hearing acuity; range of motion for neck, presence of lymphadenopathy, presence of jugular vein distention, presence of thyromegaly
Cardiovascular	Rate, rhythm, presence of murmurs, presence of rubs, presence of gallops
Pulmonary	Number of breaths per minute, respiratory effort, auscultation of lungs, presence of wheezing, presence of crackles, presence of stridor
Gastrointestinal	Appearance, tenderness, auscultation, presence of bowel sounds, hepatomegaly, splenomegaly
Genitourinary	Commonly deferred but if performed, should note lesions and discharge; costovertebral angle tenderness
Musculoskeletal	Appearance (such as muscular atrophy), range of motion, strength, and ambulation; presence of a limp or other indications of pain
Integumentary	Appearance, including lesions, rashes, bruising, presence of any surgical or injury-related scars

uncommon, with the exception of posterior cortical atrophy and progressive supranuclear palsy. Screening for vision and hearing impairments should also be performed as these may magnify any underlying cognitive impairments.

SPEECH

Deficits in speech may be noted during history-taking. Assess for difficulties in articulation, which may suggest stroke or other neurodegenerative disorders. Comprehension (the ability to follow simple and multi-step

TABLE 2.2 **Neurologic examination**

Component	Pertinent findings
Cranial nerves	Asymmetry, anosmia, extraocular movements, screen for vision and hearing impairment
Speech	Hypophonia, dysarthria, nonfluent speech, aphasia, anomia, paraphasias, syntax errors, scanning speech
Motor	Rigidity, cogwheeling, paratonia, bradykinesia; hyperreflexia, spasticity, Babinski's sign; tremor; weakness, muscle atrophy
Sensory	Polyneuropathy; deficits in light touch, vibration, proprioception, and temperature
Balance/coordination	Disequilibrium, difficulties with tandem gait, positive retropulsion test, Romberg's sign, dysmetria, dysdiadochokinesia
Posture/gait	Stooped posture, reduced arm swing; difficulties with initiation of walking and turning; wide-based gait, shuffling gait, low-steppage gait
Other	Perseveration, Luria test, apraxia, frontal release signs

requests), repetition (using simple and complex phrases), and naming (the ability to identify and name objects accurately) can be assessed individually or as part of cognitive screening tests (see Chapter 3). Deficits in comprehension, repetition, and naming may suggest Wernicke's aphasia. Assessment of naming may elicit anomia and paraphasias, which are substitutions using a generic word, a word with a similar sound (phenomic), a completely novel word (neologisms), and/or a word that has a related meaning (semantic). In fluent aphasias, patients may present with paraphasic errors with normal sentence syntax and typically good articulation. Fluent aphasias may be attributed to stroke or neurodegenerative illness localized to the temporal or parietal lobes. Listen for paucity of speech (i.e., speaking little in response to questions or only using short words or phrases), which may suggest nonfluent aphasia. Nonfluent aphasia may point to pathology near Broca's area in the frontal lobe (usually secondary to middle cerebral artery stroke or structural lesion) and may be associated with dysarthria and right hemiparesis.

The most common neurodegenerative disorders associated with an aphasic presentation are primary progressive aphasias (PPA). The semantic and nonfluent variants are typically associated with frontotemporal dementia, while the logopenic variant is associated with Alzheimer's disease. Semantic PPA is characterized by deficits in word comprehension, particularly of words that are not routinely used. Nonfluent PPA is characterized by deficits in language production, object naming, syntax errors, and word comprehension. Logopenic PPA is characterized by slowed rate of speech and impaired word retrieval and repetition, and may be accompanied by deficits in episodic memory and calculation.

MOTOR AND SENSORY EXAM

The motor and sensory exam can provide further signs to help localize lesions. Observe for fasciculations, which may suggest upper motor neuron lesions, and wasting, which may suggest lower motor neuron lesions. Abnormal movements such as tremors, bradykinesia, chorea, perseveration, myoclonus, and dystonia may be observed during the interview or upon direct examination. Assess for abnormalities in tone, such as rigidity, cogwheeling, spasticity, and paratonia. Paratonia is characterized by resistance that adjusts to the force applied (i.e., resistance increases the more rapidly the limb is moved) and may result from mesial frontal lobe pathology. Assess for power across muscle groups in the upper and lower extremities, identifying patterns of weakness and asymmetry. Also assess for reflexes, including Babinski's sign. Reflexes typically diminish with age; as such, hyperreflexia, particularly if in an asymmetric pattern, is concerning for focal pathology.

If there is concern for frontal pathology, assess for primitive reflexes (frontal release signs), such as the palmomental reflex, glabellar reflex, and/or grasp reflex. Primitive reflexes may also be observed in late stages of dementia with loss of cortical or frontal inhibition. The sensory exam should include assessment for light touch, vibration, proprioception, and temperature. Note any patterns of sensory deficits. Signs of polyneuropathy may suggest secondary causes of dementia, such as hypothyroidism, vitamin B_{12} deficiency, and diabetes.

GAIT, POSTURE, BALANCE, AND COORDINATION

While testing for balance and coordination, be wary of the patient's risk for falls. Assess the patient's gait by first asking them to walk normally, looking for any abnormalities in posture and gait not explained by known medical problems such as arthritis, polyneuropathy, or myopathies. Look for difficulties with initiation of walking and turning. Wide-based gait may suggest cerebellar pathology, normal pressure hydrocephalus, or frontal gait disorder. Frontal gait disorder is also associated with difficulty initiating movement, shuffling steps, low steppage, disequilibrium, and upright posture with preserved arm swing. Individuals with Parkinson's disease (PD) may have a shuffling gait, characterized by short strides, a narrow base, stooped posture, and reduced arm swing.

Testing tandem gait may elicit more subtle difficulties in balance and coordination. Postural stability can be affected in several neurodegenerative disorders, including PD and progressive supranuclear palsy, and can be tested using the retropulsion test. The presence of Romberg's sign may suggest dorsal column degeneration, which can be seen in vitamin B_{12} deficiency.

While completing other portions of the neurologic exam, take note of any signs of cerebellar dysfunction, such as scanning speech, nystagmus, abnormal coordination, staggering, or wide-based gait. Finger-to-nose testing may elicit dysmetria and can also be used to assess for bradykinesia and intention tremor. Test for dysdiadochokinesia with rapid alternating movements.

TESTS SPECIFIC TO FRONTAL LOBE FUNCTION

Tests aimed to elicit deficits in the frontal lobe should be used for patients where frontotemporal dementia is part of the differential. Frontal release signs, paratonia, and perseveration are consistent with frontal lobe dysfunction (described earlier in this chapter in the section on the motor and sensory exam). Perseveration may be observed in conversation (e.g., repetitive behavior, fixation on a certain topic even after it has been discussed to a point of resolution, or repetition not responsive to redirection) and also during other parts of the physical exam. For example, a patient with perseveration may continue to carry out a command even when the examiner has moved on. The Luria test is a three-step sequential task of three movements that you show the patient and ask them to repeat: making a fist, laying the hand on edge, and laying the palm down. Perseveration or failure to perform the sequential movements is abnormal. Apraxia is also associated with frontal lobe dysfunction and can be assessed by asking the patient to pretend to use a comb, write, and/or eat with a spoon.

LABORATORY TESTS

Standard initial lab tests include a complete blood count (CBC), comprehensive metabolic panel (CMP), thyroid stimulating hormone (TSH) with reflexive free thyroxine (T_4) level, fasting lipid panel, glycated hemoglobin (HbA1c) level, total vitamin D level, and vitamin B_{12} (cobalamin) level to rule out hematologic, hepatic, renal, thyroid, and cerebrovascular etiologies and vitamin deficiencies. Obtain these tests if they have not been measured within the previous year, and order them routinely at least once annually. Also obtain labs for particular positive symptoms, events, and/or suspected conditions—for example, urinalysis with urine culture (if urinary tract infection is suspected); urine drug screen (UDS) and ethyl glucuronide (EtG), acetaminophen, and salicylate levels (if substance intoxication or withdrawal is suspected); and electrocardiogram (ECG, if cardiac etiology is suspected or if the patient is currently taking antipsychotics).

Other less common lab tests for particular positive symptoms, events, and/or conditions include:

- Folate and gamma-glutamyl transferase (GGT) levels (for alcohol use disorder concerns)
- Erythrocyte sedimentation rate (ESR) and C-reactive protein (CRP) levels (for infection and/or autoimmune disorders concerns)
- Creatine phosphokinase (CPK) level (if there is prolonged immobility or if the patient is found down)
- Screening rapid plasma reagin (RPR) or Venereal Disease Research Laboratory (VDRL) tests with confirmatory *Treponema pallidum* (TPPA) or fluorescent treponemal antibody absorption (FTA-ABS) (for neurosyphilis concerns or if the patient has risk factors

including engaging in unprotected sex, having multiple sexual partners, having human immunodeficiency virus [HIV], and/or having sexual partner[s] who have tested positive for syphilis)

- Screening HIV rapid antigen/antibody test (if the patient has risk factors including engaging in unprotected sex, having multiple sexual partners, having a sexually transmitted infection, having sexual partner[s] who have tested positive for HIV, and/or sharing contaminated injection equipment)
- Autoimmune antibodies such as antinuclear antibodies (ANA) and rheumatoid factor (RF) tests (for autoimmune disorder concerns)
- Paraneoplastic antibodies (for neurologic and/or cancer concerns)
- Heavy metal screen such as arsenic, cadmium, lead, and mercury levels (for toxicity concerns)
- Cerebrospinal fluid (CSF) analysis (for meningitis, encephalitis, and/or cancer concerns; additionally, obtaining 14-3-3 protein and neuron-specific enolase for Creutzfeldt–Jakob disease [CJD] concerns)

If substance toxicity or withdrawal is suspected, obtain psychotropic and antiepileptic medication levels, if applicable, including lithium, valproic acid, carbamazepine, amitriptyline, nortriptyline, imipramine, desipramine, and doxepin. Order imaging such as chest x-ray (for infection and/or cardiopulmonary concerns). An electroencephalogram (EEG) can be ordered for seizure concerns and polysomnography or a sleep study for sleep apnea concerns. Neuroimaging such as head computed tomography (CT), magnetic resonance imaging (MRI), and positron emission tomography (PET) is also important (see Chapter 5 for detailed considerations). For many of these specific tests, consultation with the respective specialty is recommended prior to further work-up.

The exam for the patient revealed the following vitals: pulse 90, blood pressure 168/95, respiration rate 12, oxygen saturation 98%, body temperature 98.5°F, and no reported pain. A physical examination showed a fragile man with poor muscular range of motion and strength, and a slowed and unsteady gait. He had mild speech latency when asked questions. Labs showed an elevated fasting glucose of 200 and hemoglobin A1C of 7.8. Based on his history and findings, you suspect a subcortical vascular dementia and decide to order an MRI of his brain.

- A full medical examination includes vitals and a detailed physical examination.
- A full neurologic examination includes assessing cranial nerves, speech, motor and sensory abilities, balance and coordination, and posture and gait.
- Standard initial labs include a CBC, CMP, TSH with reflexive T_4 level, fasting lipid panel, HbA1c, total vitamin D level, and vitamin B_{12} level.
- Additional, more specific medical and neurological exam assessments and labs should be guided by the differential diagnosis.

Further Reading

Hategan A, Bourgeois JA, Hirsch C, Giroux C, eds. *Geriatric Psychiatry: A Case-Based Textbook*. Springer International Publishing AG; 2018.

Jacobson SA. *Laboratory Medicine in Psychiatry and Behavioral Science*. American Psychiatric Publishing; 2012.

Seraji-Bzorgzad N, Paulson H, Heidebrink J. Neurologic examination in the elderly. In: Dekosky ST, Asthana S, eds. *Handbook of Clinical Neurology: Geriatric Neurology*. Elsevier; 2019;167:73–88.

Steffens DC, Blazer DG, Thakur ME, eds. *The American Psychiatric Publishing Textbook of Geriatric Psychiatry*. 5th ed. American Psychiatric Publishing; 2015.

Summergrad P, Silbersweig DA, Muskin PR, Querques J. *Textbook of Medical Psychiatry*. American Psychiatric Association Publishing; 2020.

3 Mental status in the moment

Zelde Espinel and Elizabeth A. Crocco

A 76-year-old man was brought by his wife to the
emergency department after being involved in
a minor motor vehicle accident. The patient had
not driven for several months and had left the
house without telling his wife. When interviewed,
the patient acted relatively nonchalant about the
accident, but being distracted by people he saw
sitting in the car with him. The wife reported that
2 years ago the patient started to have episodes
in which he appeared to "blank out" for several
minutes and then return to near-normal function.
Subsequently, he began to demonstrate bilateral
hand tremor and slowness in movement. After
being prescribed risperidone, the patient rapidly
developed rigidity that became so severe that
he could not walk, and the medication had
to be discontinued. About 6 months ago, the
patient became increasingly apathetic and he
progressively withdrew from social activities that
had been a source of pleasure.

What do you do now?

In the course of the psychiatric interview for this patient, the clinician conducted a complete mental status evaluation (MSE), a critical component for the evaluation of a geriatric patient. Since geriatric patients can be poor historians due to cognitive impairment, direct observation of the patient's behaviors and verbalizations during the interview provides objective signs of illness, and the MSE provides a structure for systematically assessing the patient. The MSE is not a discrete and separate component of the patient evaluation; rather, the information that makes up the MSE is gathered throughout the entire course of the patient interview. To understand how the clinician was able to narrow the diagnosis down, the components of the MSE, as summarized in Table 3.1, will be described in more detail in this chapter.

TABLE 3.1 **MSE findings**

1.	Appearance	Adult Caucasian male, appears stated age of 76 years old, disheveled, stooped posture, masked-like facies, poor eye contact
2.	Attitude	Guarded, minimally cooperative
3.	Behavior	Psychomotor retardation
4.	Speech	Low volume, poor articulation, variable rate, aprosodia
5.	Mood	Dysphoric
6.	Affect	Flat, nonreactive
7.	Thought process	Slowed mentation, disorganized, tangential
8.	Thought content	Persecutory delusions; worthlessness, guilt, and hopelessness; negative for suicidal or homicidal ideation, preoccupations, or obsessions
9.	Perceptual disturbance	Visual hallucinations of people sitting in his car while he is driving
10.	Cognitive functioning	
	Alertness	It has fluctuated over time, with a history of "blank" episodes.

TABLE 3.1 **Continued**

	Attention	Distracted
	Orientation	Oriented to person and place, not to time
	Memory	Impairment in recall/retrieval of recent memories but not of remote events
	Concentration	Impaired
	Language	Decreased verbal fluency
	Fund of knowledge	Below baseline: unable to name past three U.S. presidents
	Executive function	Poor planning and organization of his trip outside of the house
11.	Insight	Limited insight into his condition and need for treatment
12.	Judgment	Poor judgment
13.	Motor function	
	Muscle tone	Rigidity through upper and lower extremities
	Muscle strength	Normal
	Abnormal movements	Bilateral upper extremity coarse tremor
	Gait	Abnormal, shuffling gait, bradykinesia
	Frontal release signs	None detected

COMPONENTS OF THE MSE

Appearance

Active observation of the patient is the foundation for performing the MSE. In this case, several elements of the patient's appearance provided clues to a possible neurocognitive disorder: his disheveled appearance, a stooped posture, and masked-like facies. Evaluation of appearance commences by carefully appraising the patient even before questions are asked. When describing appearance, it is important to note the patient's general degree of health, apparent age in relation to chronological age, facial expressions, eye contact, posture, grooming, and hygiene. The clinician's impression of the patient's appearance is the first indicator of psychiatric health.

Attitude

Attitude is assessed by direct observation and in the context of the relationship that develops between patient and clinician. One hallmark when describing attitude is the degree to which the patient is cooperative. The reverse may also be described: Patients may present as uncooperative, hostile, guarded, or suspicious. Lack of cooperation may be an indicator of impaired attentiveness, memory, or judgment. In the geriatric patient, attitude can be a telltale sign of neurocognitive disorders. In frontotemporal dementia, for example, patients may appear distant, cold, and indifferent. In Alzheimer's disease, patients tend to remain courteous and friendly until the late stages of the disease.

The patient's guarded attitude may reflect underlying psychosis, a common neuropsychiatric manifestation of Lewy body dementia.

Behavior

Behavior is assessed by observing the patient's physical and verbal actions and mannerisms. Degree of activity varies from psychomotor retardation to motor restlessness and disinhibition to frank agitation. Agitation is seen in all forms of dementia and is characterized by a variety of disruptive and even dangerous behaviors, including verbal or physical aggression and disinhibition. Other individuals may present as withdrawn, uncooperative, or resistant to questions or requests.

Speech

Speech impairment may affect rate, tone, volume, quantity, spontaneity, and prosody. Changes common to various forms of dementia include variable rate, poor articulation, reduced intelligibility, low volume, and impaired prosody. In the elderly, disorders of speech provide clues to underlying neurologic problems that may be caused by central or peripheral nervous system damage. Manic individuals will show rapid, pressured speech, while depressed individuals may have minimal tone and volume and offer little spontaneous speech.

Mood and Affect

A patient's emotional state is described in terms of mood and affect. While mood describes the person's internal and relatively sustained feeling state, affect is the external and rapidly changing manifestation of the internal emotional state. The relationship between mood and affect can be understood by analogy. Meteorologists often say that climate (like mood) is what you expect based on longer-term patterns, while weather (like affect) is what you get in the moment. Mood is considered the relatively stable emotional background, and affect is the emotional foreground that is changeable and influenced by mood and the external environment.

Mood is described empirically in relation to the patient's history and MSE findings. To assess mood, the clinician can ask, "How have you been feeling lately?" Common descriptors of mood include euthymic, depressed, euphoric, irritable, dysphoric, angry, or apathetic. Affect can be described along several parameters:

1. *Range*, from full to constricted
2. *Congruence* with mood
3. *Appropriateness* in relation to the content of the patient's discourse
4. *Stability*, from stable to labile
5. *Reactivity*, from reactive to nonreactive
6. *Intensity* (normal, flat, blunted, overly dramatic)

This patient's mood was dysphoric and his affect was flat and nonreactive. Depressive and anxiety symptoms may reflect common findings in Lewy body dementia. However, the evaluation of depression is made more difficult because clinicians may ascribe such depressive symptoms as blunted affect and psychomotor retardation to parkinsonian features such as bradykinesia and masked facial expression.

Thought Process

Thought process refers to the formulation, organization, and expression of thought. Because it is not possible to directly observe thought processes, these must be inferred from what the patient says. The clinician observes the flow, sequence, organization, and logic of what the patient expresses. The normal thought process is logical, goal-directed, and organized. A patient displays normal thought process when questions are answered in a manner that is direct and on point and proceeds to a logical conclusion. Disorders of thought process can manifest in several ways. Patients can display slowness of thinking called *bradyphrenia* or *bradypsychia*. Thought disorganization can be especially evident when the patient has episodes of fluctuating cognition. This includes *thought blocking*, which occurs when the patient's train of thought is disrupted mid-thought; *circumstantiality*, in which the patient pursues a winding path, infused with irrelevant details, but ultimately does return to the subject at hand; or *tangentiality*, in which the patient drifts away from the topic at hand and fails to return.

This patient showed obvious slowed thinking in interviews as there was a latency to his responses, and they were often disrupted midway through when he did respond.

Thought Content

Attentive listening, particularly during the opening moments of the session, combined with thoughtful probing, provides keys to thought content. *Delusions* are fixed, false beliefs that are not shared by others from the patient's culture; they often have a bizarre quality. In older patients, delusions may involve paranoid thoughts (e.g., of theft, harm or persecution), pathologic jealousy, somatic complaints, or misidentifications (e.g., in which the person believes that a familiar person or place is not the real or original one or has been replaced by a fake). Other notable thought content to be assessed during the MSE includes thoughts of harming oneself or others, including suicidal or homicidal ideation, intent, or plan.

The patient was developing paranoid delusions of people harming him, which are commonly seen in dementia with Lewy bodies, especially triggered by visual hallucinations of people in the environment—as was the case with him.

Perceptual Disturbances

Hallucinations are false sensory perceptions that occur in the absence of actual stimuli. They can be very vivid and at times distressing. They range from well-formed images of people, deceased relatives, animals, or insects to visions of shapes and colors. Hallucinations can be in black and white or in color. Illusions, which are misperceptions of actual stimuli, can be mistaken for hallucinations. For example, a person may perceive a chair or a lamp as a person or an animal, but the illusion corrects itself on closer visual inspection. Visual and auditory hallucinations are the most common in older individuals, especially those with various forms of dementia. Visual impairment has also been associated with hallucinations, such as in Charles Bonnet syndrome, in which a person has visual hallucinations but often recognizes them as false images.

Vivid visual hallucinations that come and go are one of the diagnostic hallmarks of dementia with Lewy bodies and often involve animals or small people (Lilliputian hallucinations) moving about the home environment.

Cognitive Functioning

Assessment of cognitive performance is important for all patients but imperative for geriatric patients, who commonly suffer from neurocognitive impairment. Cognition can be quickly assessed in the MSE using a brief cognitive screen such as the Mini–Mental State Examination (MMSE) or the Montreal Cognitive Assessment (MoCA). Cognitive screens are not used to make a specific diagnosis but rather to get a sense for the overall degree of impairment in some of the following cognitive domains.

Level of Alertness

Alertness is assessed by noting whether the patient is awake, aware, and responsive to stimuli. Fluctuations in alertness can be manifested as staring into space for long periods, daytime drowsiness, and even lethargy.

Attention and Concentration

Attention and concentration is the ability for the patient to attend to a task at hand. Concentration refers to attention that is sustained or more prolonged. Attention is assessed by abilities to perform such tasks as forward and reverse digit-span, reverse spelling, and reciting the months backwards. Patients who have impairment in attention may be easily distracted and score poorly on these tasks.

Orientation

Orientation is routinely evaluated as the patient's ability to correctly identify person, place, and time.

Memory

Assessing memory, which is defined as the ability to encode, store, recall, and remember information, is essential in the MSE for older patients. Common brief memory assessments include asking the person to recall several words or objects after several minutes, or listen to a short story and then repeat back the essential elements. Visual memory may be assessed by having the person look at a diagram and then reconstruct it several minutes later. Long-term or remote memory is assessed by asking the person to describe major past historical or personal events. Individuals with Alzheimer's disease present with severe deficits in encoding information, while those with dementia with Lewy bodies tend to show deficits in retrieval of stored information, which can be improved by providing cues. When encoding is impaired, cues are not helpful because the material is not present to be retrieved.

Language

Language should be evaluated in terms of both receptive and expressive language abilities. Receptive language is the ability to understand language in order to answer questions and follow directions and instructions. Expressive language is the ability to communicate thoughts clearly using proper grammar and vocabulary. Language is assessed by naming objects, responding to instructions, repeating a sentence, and measuring verbal fluency (i.e., producing words from a category such as food or animals, or words starting with a certain letter, such as F).

Fund of Knowledge

Fund of knowledge is explored by asking patients to provide well-known facts, such as the names of recent presidents, or other major current historical events.

Executive Function

Executive function is reflected in several skills, including planning, organization, prioritization, multitasking, reasoning, problem-solving, and inhibiting thoughts or behaviors. Several brief tests of executive function that can be administered during the MSE include the clock drawing test (the person is asked to draw the face of a clock and put on the numbers and hands to indicate a time as 11:15), trail making (drawing a line between alternating numbers and letters), and the continuous performance test (in one version, the person is asked to tap their finger each time they hear a specific letter while listening to a list of many letters and having to inhibit their response). Deficits in executive function are often related to frontal lobe injury, which is sometimes evident in frontal release signs as described in the motor exam.

The patient had noticeable fluctuations in his level of alertness over days. During the MSE he was easily distractible, which resulted in impaired attention and concentration. Memory retrieval was poor, although he did better when cued. He had decreased verbal fluency when asked to generate lists of animals. His fund of knowledge was fair, but he had a difficult time organizing his history and staying on track during the interview.

Insight

Patients with various forms of dementia and those with mania and/or delusions often display limited insight into their symptoms, which includes awareness of any underlying illness. This lack of insight can generate resistance to treatment. Such individuals are often not aware of the changes reported by informants, and may deny any changes or blame them on others.

Judgment

Judgement can be assessed by determining if the patient is making sensible and responsible decisions that help guide behavior and self-care. The clinician is also alert for the reverse: when the patient is making decisions or taking actions that may be harmful, dangerous, or illegal. Poor judgment may have consequences for the person's safety and the safety of others. One way to test judgment is to ask the patient what they would do if there was a fire or a flood in their home. Intact executive function is needed for good judgment.

On the one hand, the patient does appear to recognize that he is having changes in his mind and motor function, but he does not appreciate their true impact on his daily life. As a result, he is displaying poor judgement, as evidenced by leaving the home unexpectedly and choosing to drive despite the presence of debilitating tremor and rigidity.

The MSE will also provide a visual record of the patient's motor function, including muscle tone and strength, gait, and the presence of any abnormal movements. These are described in more detail in Chapter 2.

The MSE for this patient showed a variety of findings that were all consistent with dementia with Lewy bodies. The history and neurologic exams were all consistent with this diagnosis as well.

KEY POINTS TO REMEMBER

- Just observing the appearance, attitude, and behavior of the patient throughout the mental status interview will reveal key diagnostic indicators.
- The way in which a patient organizes and expresses their thoughts, along with the content of the thoughts, can demonstrate key symptoms of mania, depression, anxiety, and psychosis. These findings in the mental status examination can then be corroborated with the patient's reported mood and affective expression.
- With older patients in particular, a cognitive evaluation during the mental status examination is critical to identifying areas of impairment across key cognitive domains, including attention, orientation, memory, language, executive function, insight, and judgment.

Further Reading

Cummings J, Mintzer J, Brodaty H, Sano M, Banerjee S, Devanand DP, Gauthier S, Howard R, Lanctôt K, Lyketsos CG, Peskind E, Porsteinsson AP, Reich E, Sampaio C, Steffens D, Wortmann M, Zhong K; International Psychogeriatric Association. Agitation in cognitive disorders: International Psychogeriatric Association provisional consensus clinical and research definition. *Int Psychogeriatr.* 2015;27(1):7–17.

Gomperts SN. Lewy body dementias: Dementia with Lewy bodies and Parkinson disease dementia. *Continuum.* 2016;22(2 Dementia):435–463.

Harvey PD. Domains of cognition and their assessment. *Dialogues Clin Neurosci.* 2019;21(3):227–237.

McKeith IG, Boeve BF, Dickson DW, McKeith IG, Boeve BF, Dickson DW, Halliday G, Taylor J-P, Weintraub D, Aarsland D, Galvin J, Attems J, Ballard CG, Bayston A,

Beach TG, Blanc F, Bohnen N, Bonanni L, Bras J, Brundin P, et al. Diagnosis and management of dementia with Lewy bodies: Fourth consensus report of the DLB Consortium. *Neurology*. 2017;89(1):88–100.

Seraji-Bzorgzad N, Paulson H, Heidebrink J. Neurologic examination in the elderly. *Handb Clin Neurol*. 2019;167:73–88.

Trzepacz PT, Baker RW. *Psychiatric Mental Status Examination*. Oxford University Press, 1993.

4 Cognitive screens short and sweet—and when more is needed

Kelly L. Konopacki and
Sara L. Weisenbach

A 69-year-old man was referred by his primary care physician after experiencing a return of depressive symptoms following several years of remission. He and his wife also expressed concerns about memory loss and word-finding difficulty. Functionally, the patient is independent in all basic and most instrumental activities of daily living. He continues to manage his medications with minimal difficulty, although he has forgotten to take them a couple of times recently. The patient uses the internet and owns a smartphone, albeit with some trouble learning new programs and applications. Medically, the patient has a longstanding history of hypertension, hyperlipidemia, and hypothyroidism, which have been well controlled with medication. Family history is remarkable for dementia of unknown etiology in his mother.

What do you do now?

Given that cognitive changes are not always readily apparent to the care provider, the patient, or the patient's care partners, cognitive screenings should ideally be performed annually for all patients aged 65 and older. In this case, there is also the presence of a cognitive complaint and a family history of dementia. Which screening measure should you use, and how do you administer and score it and interpret the patient's performance?

It is imperative to use reliable and valid screening methods with patients at risk for cognitive decline. The most commonly used instruments are listed in Table 4.1. Although these scales have generally good validation and reliability, the identification of cognitive decline during earlier stages of a neurodegenerative process may be impeded by less-than-perfect sensitivity (proportion of actual positives identified as positive) and specificity (proportion of actual negatives identified as negative). Several factors can further limit their accuracy.

For example, performance on a cognitive screen reflects a snapshot of the patient's abilities, as opposed to a reflection of longitudinal change. A patient's performance may be impacted by a multitude of transient variables (e.g., fatigue, medications, mood, effort, sleep) and therefore should not be used to diagnose a neurocognitive disorder. Cognitive screens typically include only one or two items aimed at assessing a particular aspect/domain of cognition (e.g., memory). As a result, the patient's performance on the screen is not necessarily a reliable reflection of their actual abilities in the measured domain. For individuals with high educational attainment and/or greater cognitive reserve, performance in the "normal" range may not rule out true cognitive decline.

To optimize the data gained from these screens, administration should be completed in a standardized manner. Ideally, the patient and examiner are the only people in the room during administration in order to minimize factors that might impact performance (e.g., distraction, third-party observer effects). The patient's comfort with the English language should be considered when administering tools that were developed and normed in English-speaking samples. Notably, there are cognitive screening instruments that have been translated into other languages and normed using data from native speakers.

In the case presented, suppose you decide to administer the Montreal Cognitive Assessment (MoCA) and the patient performed in the normal

TABLE 4.1 Commonly used cognitive screening measures

Test	Description	Cut-off	Sensitivity	Specificity
Montreal Cognitive Assessment (MoCA)	30-point comprehensive screen including tests of executive function such as trail making and clock drawing	<26	90% (MCI)	87% (MCI)
6-Item Screen	Orientation items and 3-item recall	<4	88.7% (dementia)	88% (dementia)
Mini-Cog	3-item recall plus clock drawing test	<3	76–99% (dementia)	83–93% (dementia)
Clock drawing test (CLOX)	Directed clock-drawing and clock reproduction	Varies with version	89% (Alzheimer's)	91% (Alzheimer's)
Category fluency	60-second task to list words or items in a category (e.g., starting with a specific letter, or animal names)	<17	88% (Alzheimer's)	96% (Alzheimer's)
Mini–Mental State Examination (MMSE)	30-point semi-comprehensive screen. which lacks specific items to assess executive function	<24	85% (dementia)	90% (dementia)
St. Louis Mental Status Exam (SLUMS)	30-point comprehensive screen which includes tests of executive function	<27		

range, scoring 26 out 30 points total. Given the patient's "normal" score, should you dismiss concerns of cognitive decline? An important consideration in this case is the patient's high level of educational attainment (i.e., a master's degree), so a "normal" performance on this or other screens may still represent a significant decline from baseline. In this and many other cases, complaints of memory loss are typical among older adults with depression. In addition, depression is a known risk factor for dementia and sometimes represents an initial sign of a neurodegenerative condition. What do you do now?

With this knowledge in mind, you could increase the dosage of his antidepressants in order to reduce his depressive and anxious symptoms and potentially improve his cognition, and then repeat the screen in 8 weeks. On follow-up, the patient's mood has noticeably improved; however, when you readminister the MoCA using an alternate form (to minimize practice effects), his score dropped by 2 points, to 24 out of 30. Now what do you do?

At this point, cognitive problems are evident by self-report and informant report and an objective cognitive screening. You consider potentially reversible causes (i.e., active state of depression) and determine that an evaluation would clarify whether the patient is experiencing a neurodegenerative process. You recommend a referral for a more comprehensive neuropsychological evaluation to assess for possible mild cognitive impairment (MCI) or dementia, as a diagnosis will assist both patient and care providers in treatment and care planning, as well as potential participation in clinical trials.

NEUROPSYCHOLOGICAL EVALUATION

Neuropsychology is the study of brain–behavior relationships, and neuropsychological evaluations aim to assess a variety of cognitive abilities and to understand the biologic and functional causes of dysfunction to improve patient and disease management and treatment. A neuropsychological evaluation is most beneficial when (a) reversible causes of cognitive decline have been ruled out; (b) diagnostic clarity is needed; and/or (c) the rate and extent of cognitive and functional changes require clarification. A referral to neuropsychology should clearly delineate the purpose of the evaluation and what you hope to learn, and the evaluation should be conducted by a clinical neuropsychologist. It typically begins with an information-gathering interview with the patient and corroborating informant. The interview covers the onset, trajectory, and nuances of cognitive changes, functional abilities, and other background information (e.g., educational and occupational history) to assist in contextualizing the patient's cognition and functional changes. Based on the information collected, the neuropsychologist develops a battery of tests that examine multiple aspects of cognition (Table 4.2) and that will take approximately 2 to 4 hours to administer. Throughout the evaluation, the neuropsychologist also makes behavioral observations (e.g., orientation, speech/language skills, affect, motor functioning). After the testing is completed, the performances are scored and the neuropsychologist interprets the results based upon normative data that reflect age and sometimes education, race, and sex. The neuropsychologist then looks for specific patterns of performance or scores consistent with certain disorders or diseases and develops a case conceptualization based on the elements of the evaluation described earlier. The test battery may also include embedded tests of effort, which help identify whether there may be a volitional element to underperformance.

In the case presented, the neuropsychologist concluded that the patient's cognitive profile was most consistent with the early stages of a neurodegenerative disorder, likely of the Alzheimer's type, but potentially mixed with vascular etiology. How did the neuropsychologist come to this conclusion? Cognition among older adults with depression is often lower across multiple domains than their never-depressed same-age peers. While this is certainly true in this case, the severity of the patient's memory deficits was beyond what is expected from the effects of late-life depression alone. And while mood is likely exacerbating his cognitive difficulties, it is unlikely to be the sole or primary cause of his cognitive decline. However, patterns of performance within his neurocognitive profile were consistent with that commonly seen in the early stages of Alzheimer's disease (i.e., most notable weaknesses in episodic memory, semantic verbal fluency, and naming). The neuropsychologist concluded that vascular etiology may also be a contributing factor given his history of vascular-related health conditions. In the end, the patient met formal criteria for multi-domain amnestic MCI because he performed significantly below same-age peers on memory tasks,

TABLE 4.2 **Cognitive domains commonly examined by a neuropsychological evaluation**

Cognitive domain/ construct	Brief description	Examples of methods to assess cognitive construct
Global cognitive function	General estimate of overall cognitive ability	Intelligence quotient/ summation of verbal, visuospatial, processing speed, and working memory skills
Attention and concentration	Simple and sustained attention/focus	Digit span repetition/ sequencing, mental arithmetic, and serial 7s
Processing speed	Speed at which a person completes a mental task and/or understands/reacts to information	Speeded visual scanning, target detection, hand–eye coordination
Psychomotor functioning and speed/dexterity	Relationship between cognitive processes and motor movements (e.g., fine motor movements/ coordination)	Speed and accuracy of placing pegs in pegboard, ability to perform skilled tasks on command or by imitation and use objects appropriately
Speech and language	Speech (articulation, rate, rhythm, volume) and receptive and expressive language skills (e.g., comprehension and production)	Vocabulary; ability to name objects, follow simple and multistep instructions, describe a scene/picture
Visuospatial and visuoconstructional skills	Visual perception and construction	Ability to construct designs using blocks, draw/copy designs, solve visual puzzles, detect angles of lines

TABLE 4.2 **Continued**

Cognitive domain/ construct	Brief description	Examples of methods to assess cognitive construct
Learning and memory	Encoding/registration, storage/consolidation, and retrieval of knowledge	Word-list (rote) verbal learning and recall and recognition memory, immediate and delayed recall and recognition of stories (contextual), immediate and delayed recall and recognition of geometric designs and spatial location
Working memory and executive functioning	Working memory, mental flexibility/ multitasking, planning/ organization, inhibition, problem-solving	Ability to switch between two tasks, inhibiting a habitual response (Stroop), drawing a complex figure, verbal fluency, abstract reasoning, solving novel problems
Mood/emotional functioning	Depression, anxiety, etc.	Self and informant questionnaires measuring mood symptoms
Functional skills	Basic and instrumental activities of daily living	Ability to dress, feed, bathe self, manage finances, drive, maintain a healthy living environment

aspects of executive functioning, expressive language, and processing speed. He did *not* meet criteria for dementia because he remained independent for basic and instrumental activities of daily living.

After the testing and interpretation was completed, the neuropsychologist met with the patient and his wife for a feedback session during which the results, diagnostic impressions, prognosis, and treatment recommendations were discussed. Some of the recommendations provided in this case included continued psychiatric treatment of anxiety and depression, a formal driving evaluation (due to executive dysfunction), a repeat neuropsychological evaluation in 12 to 18 months in order to monitor for potential progression of cognitive decline, use of memory aids (e.g., a pocket notebook to jot down quick reminders, alarms to remind him to take his medications, and a planner to remind him of future appointments), and a referral to social work to assist with future care-planning needs. The feedback session also provided the patient and his wife with the opportunity to ask the neuropsychologist questions. The neuropsychologist shared these findings with the requesting clinician, who in turn considered sending the patient for magnetic resonance imaging (MRI) of his brain to help quantify potential small-vessel cerebrovascular disease.

KEY POINTS TO REMEMBER

- Cognitive screening should be conducted at least annually among adults aged 65 years and older, and when there is observation or report of cognitive change.
- Cognitive screening should utilize an instrument that is reliable, valid, sensitive, specific, and standardized. Such instruments should not be used for diagnostic purposes.
- Comprehensive neuropsychological evaluation can provide diagnostic clarity and guidance for treatment planning.

Further Reading

Abd Razak MA, Ahmad NA, Chan YY, Mohamad Kasim N, Abdul Ghani MKA, Omar M, Abd Aziz FA, Jamaluddin R. Validity of screening tools for dementia and mild cognitive impairment among the elderly in primary health care: A systematic review. *Public Health*. 2019;169:84–92.

Burke SL, Grudzien A, Burgess A, Rodriguez MJ, Rivera Y, Lowenstein D. The utility of cognitive screeners in the detection of dementia spectrum disorders in Spanish-speaking populations. *J Geriatr Psychiatry Neurol*. 2021;34(2):102–118.

Cordell CB, Borson S, Boustani M, Chodosh J, Reuben D, Verghese J, Thies W, Fried LB; Medicare Detection of Cognitive Impairment Workgroup. Alzheimer's Association recommendations for operationalizing the detection of cognitive impairment during the Medicare Annual Wellness Visit in a primary care setting. *Alzheimers Dement*. 2013;9(2):141–150.

5 A picture worth a thousand words

Brandon Yarns and Aaron Greene

A 62-year-old male presents to a memory clinic with significant social disengagement and "bumping into things" for an indeterminate amount of time. His wife has taken over all driving, cooking, shopping, and management of his medications. The review of systems is otherwise negative. He endorses a family history of elderly relatives being placed in long-term care facilities; however, he does not know their diagnoses. His Montreal Cognitive Assessment (MoCA) score in clinic is 19/30, with deficits in visuospatial, executive function, attention, delayed recall, and orientation. Basic laboratory tests were unremarkable. The patient is visibly disengaged during the interview and irritable when asked questions.

What do you do now?

Given this patient's unusual constellation of symptoms with an unknown onset and course and relatively young age, a broad differential diagnosis is needed. Delirium is unlikely since he has not had any recent illnesses, and the review of systems and laboratory test results are unremarkable. Based on his functional impairment, there is concern for an underlying major neurocognitive disorder (dementia) with a wide differential diagnosis, including Alzheimer's disease (AD) with visuospatial variant, frontotemporal dementia (FTD), dementia with Lewy bodies (DLB), vascular dementia, or even a rarer subtype such as Creutzfeldt–Jakob disease. Less likely but also possible is subdural hematoma (even without a known recent head injury) or tumor. While AD is the most common type of neurodegenerative dementia and has a lifetime prevalence that increases up to over 50% by age 85, one should always suspect early-onset AD when the symptomatic picture occurs before age 65. FTD generally presents between the ages of 40 and 60 years and may manifest as several variant forms. Further neuroimaging studies may help clarify his diagnosis.

USING BIOMARKERS AND NEUROIMAGING FOR DEMENTIA DIAGNOSIS

Guidelines for the diagnosis of dementia vary in the degree that they emphasize incorporating biomarkers, such as neuroimaging studies, into diagnostic criteria, with most continuing to broadly favor exclusively clinical diagnoses that rely on a history of cognitive symptoms and functional impairment. For instance, the guidelines for minor and major neurocognitive disorders in the fifth edition of the American Psychiatric Association's *Diagnostic and Statistical Manual of Mental Disorders* (DSM-5) do not require or suggest any biomarker studies to establish these diagnoses, except in the case of vascular dementia. The 2014 International Workgroup Guidelines require the presence of clinical symptoms and biomarkers (either amyloid positron emission tomography [PET] or both cerebrospinal fluid [CSF] amyloid beta [Aβ] and tau), and the 2011 National Institute on Aging/Alzheimer's Association (NIA-AA) guidelines provide information on how biomarkers can be used to support a diagnosis of AD in individuals already displaying symptoms. However, the 2001 American Academy of

Neurology AD diagnostic guidelines suggest structural imaging, such as magnetic resonance imaging (MRI), for all dementia work-ups.

Obtaining neuroimaging can help to establish an accurate diagnosis and hence determine the best management approaches. For instance, acetylcholinesterase inhibitors are considered helpful for AD and DLB but less helpful for vascular dementia or FTD. In recent years, there have been several advancements in neuroimaging options related to AD, particularly the discovery of qualitative and quantitative molecular imaging techniques that allow for the visualization of abnormal deposition of brain Aβ and tau. Currently, access to these techniques remains limited mostly to clinical trials, with clinical applications not yet well established. However, as neuroimaging techniques and treatments for AD and other forms of dementia continue to improve, neuroimaging will likely become increasingly important in clinical practice to establish accurate diagnoses and perhaps even to monitor response to treatment, especially if there is approval of disease-modifying treatments for AD.

STRUCTURAL IMAGING

Structural imaging refers to anatomic MRI or computed tomography (CT). CT is considered the optimal modality to evaluate acute, subacute, or chronic bleeding, such as a subdural hematoma. For the assessment of patients with cognitive decline suggestive of a neurodegenerative process, MRI is regarded as superior to CT, but some patients cannot undergo MRI scanning due to having foreign metal in their body or due to claustrophobia. In research studies, qualitative estimates of medial temporal lobe (MTL) atrophy on CT correlate with similar MRI findings and autopsy-proven AD, so CT may be suitable for those who cannot undergo MRI. In clinical practice, assessment of CT or MRI scans by radiologists is usually qualitative rather than quantitative. Some semi-quantitative scales have been developed for clinical practice to assess MTL atrophy in cases of suspected AD.

The American Academy of Neurology recommends obtaining structural imaging one time for the work-up of any patient with cognitive impairment, and its use is increasingly common. Several MRI sequences are usually used to assess possible neurodegenerative processes. T1-weighted sequences show cerebrospinal fluid (CSF) as dark and gray matter as relatively darker than white matter and are best for visualizing anatomy. T2-weighted sequences show CSF as bright and gray matter as relatively brighter than white matter. FLAIR is a variant of T2 in which CSF is shown as dark; FLAIR is useful for visualizing hemosiderin deposition and hyperintensities such as white matter disease. Diffusion-weighted imaging (DWI) is a measurement of the rate of diffusion (also known as random Brownian motion) of water molecules within tissues. These imaging techniques are summarized in Table 5.1.

Most clinicians will find themselves at least once in their career facing the dilemma of whether to order brain imaging with or without contrast. Non-contrast brain imaging, in particular MRI, is able to uncover anatomic pathologies that may be associated with neurocognitive impairment such as mass lesions/mass effects, strokes, abscesses, normal pressure hydrocephalus, and regions of atrophy. Iodine and barium sulfate–based compounds are the contrast agents used most often with CT, while gadolinium is most commonly used with MRI. Brain imaging with contrast is an important

TABLE 5.1 **MRI imaging modalities**

Modality	When it is used	How do they appear?
T1*	Best for visualizing anatomy	CSF is dark, and gray matter is darker than white matter.
T2*	White matter disease	CSF is bright, and gray matter is lighter than white matter.
FLAIR	Visualizing bleeds (hemosiderin) and white matter disease	Variant of T2 with spinal fluid as dark
DWI	Acute ischemic stroke	Bright
Gadolinium	With T1, used for vascular structures (tumors), breakdown in blood–brain barrier (abscesses), multiple sclerosis	Bright

*T1 and T2 refer to different "timing" sequences when obtaining the images.

tool for enhancing visualization of a subset of pathologies that can present with neurocognitive impairments such as infection, metastatic disease, carotid stenosis, and cranial nerve lesions, which are usually present along with associated clinical signs and symptoms. For patients being assessed for acute stroke, contrast should be avoided in case hemorrhaging is present and for patients seen for post-stroke monitoring.

Absolute contraindications to MRI include implanted or embedded magnetic metal anywhere in the body such as a cardiac pacemaker or defibrillator, shrapnel from welding, hearing aids, magnetic dental implants, as well as jewelry. Silicone, dental fillings, and dental implants are usually safe for MRI because most are made with titanium. While pure titanium implants are safe, caution needs to be taken for the possibility of an implant being a titanium alloy, as they may contain ferromagnetic materials that could interact magnetically and/or materials that may react thermodynamically, causing significant heating. If in question, a preliminary X-ray can be performed to screen for the presence of foreign metal in the body. Relative contraindications include a joint replacement or prosthesis, artery or airway stents, recent tattoo or colonoscopy, and programmable shunts. Contraindications to MRI with contrast include all of those for MRI without contrast as well as previous adverse reaction to gadolinium, estimated glomerular filtration rate below 30 mL/min/1.73 m^2, patients on dialysis, history of renal disease, and having received a dose of contrast within the past 24 hours. Other relative contraindications include how well the patient is able to tolerate lying still in the machine and breathing while lying down, and how well the patient can fit into the machine. Many systems have screening measures in place to ensure appropriate use of imaging techniques; however, if in question, it is appropriate to consult the performing radiology department for further guidance.

For patient with severe claustrophobia there are two options. First, you can sedate the patient with a short-acting benzodiazepine. Alternatively, you could use an "open MRI" machine, which has a much larger bore that doesn't feel so enclosing. The limitations of open MRI compared to standard machines are that the image quality and diagnostic accuracy are lower due to the lower-strength magnets used, certain body parts cannot easily be placed in the necessary area to obtain usable images, and they take longer to obtain images.

Traditionally, structural imaging has been used to exclude non-neurodegenerative causes of impaired cognition, including brain tumors, hydrocephalus, abscesses, strokes, or hemorrhage. After excluding structural lesions, the next step is to look for global cerebral atrophy, which, if present, may provide nonspecific evidence of a neurodegenerative process. After investigating global cerebral atrophy, assess for regional patterns of atrophy, which may be more suggestive of specific diagnoses. However, even classic patterns of regional atrophy on structural imaging should be regarded as nonspecific and must be correlated with clinical data.

The classic pattern of atrophy that suggests AD is cortical loss in the parietal and temporal lobes with notable sparing of the sensorimotor strip. Atrophy is often especially noted in the MTL and the precuneus, with the earliest atrophy thought to manifest in the MTL. Thus, the imaging protocol for AD should include a T1-weighted coronal sequence perpendicular to the long axis of the hippocampus, which is thought to be the best sequence and orientation to assess MTL atrophy. Notably, many studies show that white matter disease is common in normal aging and in patients with AD, and therefore its presence does not necessarily suggest that vascular dementia is the sole diagnosis. A qualitative estimate of the amount of white matter disease can be useful in determining whether this is a manifestation of normal aging or suggestive of dementia.

In FTD, the classic pattern of atrophy is cortical loss in the anterior frontal and temporal lobes with sparing of the parietal and occipital lobes. Hippocampal atrophy may be seen in FTD. Therefore, visualization of the hippocampus must be in relation to other structures. In DLB, the classic pattern of atrophy is cortical loss in the occipital lobes with sparing of the posterior cingulate gyrus, referred to as the "cingulate island sign." Vascular dementia may display abnormalities asymmetrically and anywhere there has been a vascular insult. In the case of rapidly progressive dementia, T2-weighted hyperintensities in the basal ganglia and cortex and diffusion restriction on DWI are suggestive of Creutzfeldt–Jakob disease.

FLUORODEOXYGLUCOSE (FDG) PET

Neurogenerative diseases produce damage and diminished function in cerebral tissues that result in alterations of their normal metabolism. This hypometabolism can be visualized using fluorine 18 (^{18}F) fluorodeoxyglucose (FDG) PET. Classic patterns of FDG PET hypometabolism are considered characteristic of specific degenerative diseases, which can be useful when MRI alone does not demonstrate a classic pattern suggestive of a diagnosis. The classic FDG PET pattern in AD is reductions in posterior cingulate, parietal, temporal, prefrontal, and whole-brain cerebral metabolic rates for glucose. These changes are progressive and correlate with disease severity. In FTD, the classic pattern of hypometabolism is cortical reduction in the anterior frontal and temporal lobes with sparing of the parietal and occipital lobes. FDG PET is considered particularly useful in differentiating FTD from AD.

FDG PET may also be considered when symptoms are unusual or present diagnostic difficulties. In one study, agreement between FDG PET and neuropathologic diagnosis was between 75% and 90% using six raters and better than the correlation between clinical examination and neuropathologic diagnosis (75% to 80%). FGD PET may also be useful in differentiating neurologic disease from psychiatric and drug-induced causes of behavioral and cognitive dysfunction. FDG PET scans are frequently abnormal even when symptoms of neurologic disease are very mild and can be of clinical utility in establishing a likely, though nonspecific, neurodegenerative basis for mild symptoms of memory loss and cognitive dysfunction.

AMYLOID PET

While the clinical diagnosis of AD involves an evaluation of cognitive symptoms and functional impairment, it has long been known that histopathologically the disease is characterized by the accumulation of Aβ plaques and misfolded tau-protein neurofibrillary tangles. There are now several radiotracers that allow for visualization of abnormal amyloid aggregation using PET imaging. The Society of Nuclear Medicine and Molecular Imaging and the Alzheimer's Association developed an Amyloid Imaging Task Force (AIT) that proposed criteria for the use of amyloid PET in clinical practice. The AIT suggested that amyloid brain imaging should only be used when:

- Patients have a cognitive complaint and objectively confirmed impairment

- The diagnosis of AD remains uncertain after a comprehensive evaluation by a dementia expert
- The presence or absence of amyloid would increase the certainty of the diagnosis and alter the treatment plan.

This would include patients with persistent or progressive unexplained mild cognitive impairment, atypical presentations (such as prominent language deficits, visuospatial deficits, or executive dysfunction without prominent memory impairment) who meet criteria for AD, and development of a progressive dementia at an unusually early age of onset, such as less than 65 years. However, the AIT does not recommend amyloid PET for patients who are over age 65 years who meet the standard definitions and tests for AD or in asymptomatic patients or patients with a cognitive complaint that has not been objectively confirmed, such as patients requesting amyloid PET solely because of a family history of dementia or risk factors such as the *ApoE-4* gene.

Amyloid PET imaging (and tau imaging, described shortly) can yield either qualitative or quantitative reports. In either case, scans should be interpreted by an imaging expert, such as a nuclear medicine specialist or radiologist with specific training. Qualitative interpretation relies on the visual comparison of signal intensity in brain regions in the cortex compared to the cerebellum, which is expected to have uptake. Quantitative interpretation calculates standard uptake value ratios (SUVr) in the cortex compared to the cerebellum. A priori threshold SUVr values, such as SUVr ≥ 1.17 in some guidelines, can be used as cut-offs for positive and negative scans. In 2018, a new research framework for AD was established by the NIA-AA that highlights how AD always involves amyloid plaque deposition in the brain. However, the pattern of Aβ deposition and the significance of amyloid burden with regard to clinical symptoms is still not well understood. Thus, both the NIA-AA and AIT groups suggest amyloid imaging is not useful for monitoring the severity of AD.

TAU PET

Only recently has a radiotracer been developed that binds specifically to intracellular and extracellular tau proteins. As of this writing, tau-based PET has limited access in clinical practice but is being used primarily in research settings. Abnormal tau proteins are found in the histopathology of AD and FTD. The accumulation of the radiotracer should correspond to the pathologic areas, including the hippocampus and precuneus for AD and the frontal and temporal lobes for FTD. Diffuse uptake along the gray–white junction may be found in chronic traumatic encephalopathy, and uptake may also be present in corticobasal degeneration and progressive supranuclear palsy. Tau uptake should not be present in DLB or PD. A recent study out of the University of California at San Francisco, published in *Science Translational Medicine*, indicated that tau-protein "tangles" reliably predicted the location of brain atrophy in AD patients 1 year out, whereas the location of amyloid deposits was of little value in predicting future damage. These promising findings suggest that tau PET may be of clinical utility in the future.

SPECT

As an alternative to FDG PET, SPECT imaging is less widely available and has fewer radiotracer ligands and lower resolution. Therefore, its potential clinical applicability may be lower than that of FDG PET. The one case where SPECT should be used is in areas of diagnostic uncertainty between AD and DLB or another parkinsonian syndrome. These are cases where cognitive symptoms are present along with parkinsonian (movement disorder) symptoms or visual symptoms, such as visual hallucinations. In this case, iodine 123 (^{123}I) ioflupane SPECT, commonly known as the DaTscan (GE Healthcare), can be used. This agent binds to the dopamine transporters located in the striatum. The normal distribution has a comma-shaped appearance in the caudate head and putamen. However, with parkinsonian pathology, there is reduced uptake in the putamen that results in the appearance of a "period" and can sometimes progress to a nearly complete loss of uptake.

In this patient's case, you order a brain MRI without contrast (including T1- and T2-weighted images and DWI), which shows no mass lesions or bleeding, mild to moderate diffuse atrophy in excess of what would be expected for his age, and mild white matter disease. Because this does not point to a specific diagnosis, you decide to order FDG PET, which shows hypometabolism in the temporal and parietal lobes with normal metabolism in the sensorimotor strip.

Although the patient may have met AIT criteria to order amyloid PET due to his age (<65 years) and his somewhat atypical presenting symptoms, an FDG PET was ordered and showed a classic pattern suggestive of AD. As a result, you decide no further imaging studies are needed, start the patient on an ace- tylcholinesterase inhibitor, and provide psychoeducation to him and his family regarding behavioral management of his irritability. Three months later, the patient and his wife report reduced irritability and mild improvements in his functioning, as he is now able to help his wife with looking for items while shop- ping and with washing the dishes.

KEY POINTS TO REMEMBER

- Structural imaging is clinically useful for identifying or ruling out non-neurodegenerative causes of cognitive dysfunction, which may or may not be reversible, such as vascular pathology, abscesses, and mass lesions. T1- and T2-weighted MRI without contrast are commonly used imaging techniques for the initial work-up of dementia, while DWI and other sequences can be useful for ruling out other potential causes of neurocognitive impairment when there is clinical suspicion.
- While there are specific patterns of atrophy that are representative of distinct variants of neurodegenerative disease, they are often not diagnostically definitive, are less prevalent than nonspecific findings, and may be difficult to identify without adequate comparative data.
- Molecular imaging including FDG PET and amyloid or tau PET can provide qualitative or quantitative results and is clinically useful for corroborating or ruling out suspected underlying neurodegenerative processes, given that the appropriate type of scan and ligand are chosen.

Further Reading

Vernooij MW, van Buchem MA. Neuroimaging in dementia. In: Hodler J, Kubik-Huch RA, von Schulthess GK, eds. *Diseases of the Brain, Head and Neck, Spine 2020– 2023: Diagnostic Imaging.* Springer; 2020:131–142. https://www.springer.com/gp/book/9783030384890

Patel KP, Wymer DT, Bhatia VK, Duara R, Rajadhyaksha CD. Multimodality imaging of dementia: Clinical importance and role of integrated anatomic and molecular imaging. *Radiographics.* 2020;40(1):200–222.

Staffaroni AM, Ehali FM, McDermott D, Morton K, Karageorgiou E, Sacco S, Paoletti M, Caverzasi E, Hess CP, Rosen HJ, Geschwind MD. Neuroimaging in dementia. *Semin Neurol.* 2017;37(5):510–537.

6   What's normal and what's not? Putting it all together

Saumil Dholakia, Sophiya Benjamin, and Joanne Ho

A 69-year-old retired lawyer with a history of hypertension, dyslipidemia, diabetes, and depression presents with at least 1 year of self-reported forgetfulness. He is disappointed to have mixed up the dates of several social events and he increasingly writes things down to keep track of appointments and tasks. His daughter notes that he is otherwise independent in caring for himself. However, she notices that he has "slowed down" when walking, and seems more depressed since his spouse's sudden death 1 year ago. On a brief mental status exam, he acknowledges feeling lonely and isolated with a general lack of drive. He scores 27 out of 30 on the Mini–Mental State Examination (MMSE), losing 3 points in short-term recall of three words. He expresses anxiety about ending up like his mother, whose dementia started at age 83 years.

What do you do now?

Are the memory changes experienced by this patient due to normal aging and life-stage stressors, mild cognitive impairment (MCI), or a major neurocognitive disorder (MNCD)? Differentiating amnestic changes of MCI from those intrinsic to normal aging is crucial: Individuals with MCI have dementia progression rates of around 10% to 12% per year as compared to population incidence figures in normal older adults of 1% to 2% per year. Approaching the wide differential diagnosis of subjective cognitive impairment requires a systematic approach. In addition to neurodegenerative processes that result in MNCDs, medical factors including vascular disease, head trauma, family history, previous delirium, structural central nervous system lesions, metabolic disease, and medications may contribute to or exacerbate the deficits. Mental illnesses that may affect memory include recurrent or chronic mood disorders and late-onset schizophrenia spectrum disorders. Putting all this together, one helpful way to clarify the differential diagnosis of cognitive impairment is referred to as the 4Ds Approach: Diagnosis, Drugs, Dysfunction in cognitive domains, and Dementia subtype and staging.

DIAGNOSIS

Cognitive impairment may be the result of a range of medical and psychiatric disorders (Table 6.1) that may occur in isolation but more commonly occur in combination. Clarifying the timing of symptoms and identifying risk or protective factors from the medical history is informative for diagnosis, management, and prognosis. Use of a general mnemonic such as "VINDICATE" to systematically approach cognitive impairment may be of assistance.

A lack of emotional drive or a recent significant loss and a history of depression points toward depression as a possible etiology in this case. This could be clarified by using screening tools such as the Geriatric Depression Scale (GDS-15) or the Patient Health Questionnaire (PHQ-9) in people with MCI and the Cornell Scale of Depression in Dementia in people with moderate to severe cognitive impairment to help establish the nature and severity of depression. Because symptoms of reversible cognitive impairment associated with depression, also known as pseudodementia, improve with treatment, it is important to capture this diagnosis in all patients presenting with memory complaints.

TABLE 6.1 **Differential diagnosis for medical illnesses causing cognitive impairment**

Physical illness	Examples
Vascular	Vascular dementia, hemorrhagic or ischemic stroke, cerebral sinus venous thrombosis
Infection	Viral, bacterial, fungal, prion infections
Neoplasm	Central nervous system primary or secondary malignancy, paraneoplastic encephalitis
Drugs	Toxicity, intoxication or withdrawal
Degenerative	Major neurocognitive disorder (Alzheimer's disease, Parkinson's disease dementia, Lewy body dementia, frontotemporal dementia)
Iatrogenic	Medications
Congenital	Huntington's disease, Alzheimer's disease associated with presenilin gene mutations or trisomy 21, Wilson's disease
Autoimmune	Vasculitis, systemic lupus erythematosus, Hashimoto's encephalopathy
Trauma	Traumatic brain injury with bleeding, chronic traumatic encephalopathy, delirium, seizure
Endocrine/metabolic	Thyroid dysfunction, renal disease, hypoxia, hypercarbia (obstructive sleep apnea, chronic obstructive lung disease), hyperglycemia, electrolyte disturbances (hyponatremia, hypernatremia, hypercalcemia), heavy metals

Understanding changes in gait, mobility, and movement can also provide insight into the diagnosis of cognitive impairment. For example, changes in gait may be an early symptom of several forms of dementia, especially when there is also emerging parkinsonism (e.g., tremor, rigidity, akinesia, stooped posture). The differential diagnosis will include Parkinson's disease, Lewy body dementia, progressive supranuclear palsy, corticobasilar degeneration, normal pressure hydrocephalus, and vascular dementia associated with damage to the basal ganglia.

A review of systems should include questions about sleep, appetite, constitutional symptoms, and bladder or bowel symptoms. For example, constipation, low energy, and heat intolerance may suggest hypothyroidism. The presence of fever, night sweats, and weight loss might be seen with malignancy or autoimmune disorders. Standard investigations can identify infection, autoimmune, endocrine, or metabolic causes. Neuroimaging may help rule out reversible and/or structural causes of cognitive impairment, particularly in this patient who has vascular risk factors.

DRUGS

Medication reconciliation is an important component of any encounter with a patient experiencing cognitive impairment. Medications that reduce acetylcholine directly or indirectly through increased dopaminergic, serotoninergic, and norepinephrinergic activity or increased GABAergic and glutamatergic transmission contribute to cognitive dysfunction. These are outlined in Table 6.2.

Additional history in this case reveals no history suggestive of an alcohol, smoking, or substance use disorder. There is no history of falls or head trauma. His medications include regular antidiabetic and antihypertensive agents as well as a benzodiazepine for sleep. His physical examination is unremarkable aside from a slow and overly cautious gait. While you optimize his other medications, you discuss and systematically taper the benzodiazepine and substitute a safer supplement along coupled with nonpharmacologic approaches to improve his sleep.

DYSFUNCTION IN COGNITIVE DOMAINS

The patient's increasing reliance on lists and calendars as memory aids and new frustration in social gatherings indicate memory deficits and new-onset executive dysfunction, respectively. His function is relatively preserved; therefore, this weighs in favor of an MCI diagnosis at this time. Assigning diagnostic weights to deficits in cognitive domains helps determine if the individual's cognitive function is normal for age and life stage or is compatible with a diagnosis of MCI. Table 6.3 illustrates clinical insights that aid in evaluating all six cognitive domains.

TABLE 6.2 **Medications causing cognitive impairment**

Medications	Common examples
Anticholinergic	Dimenhydrinate, diphenhydramine, tricyclic antidepressants, benztropine, antiemetics (e.g., prochlorperazine, dimenhydrinate), overactive bladder medications (e.g., oxybutynin, tolterodine), carbamazepine, paroxetine
Sedative–hypnotics	Benzodiazepine and non-benzodiazepine benzodiazepine receptor agonists (zopiclone, zolpidem), barbiturates
Analgesics	Opioids, tramadol, gabapentinoids
Glucocorticoids	Acute or chronic use of glucocorticoids
Dopaminergic medications	Excess in levodopa, pramipexole, bupropion, illicit drugs (e.g., cocaine)
Natural health products	Valerian, cannabis-derived products
Serotonergic medications	Excess in antidepressants, lithium, monoamine oxidase inhibitors, illicit drugs (e.g., cocaine, MDMA)
Recreational substances (with multiple effects on neurotransmitters)	Cannabis and cannabis-derived products, amphetamines, alcohol, cocaine

How much do memory-screening tests add to diagnostic weights? Once a clinical diagnosis of MCI is made, screening office memory tests aid in documenting the nature and severity of memory dysfunctions (also see Chapter 4). Psychometric screening instruments, such as the MMSE and the Montreal Cognitive Assessment (MoCA), can also track changes in cognitive functioning over time and the response to therapeutic agents (see Chapter 4). However, using any screening test with one single cut-off score to define cognitive impairment should be done in conjunction with robust collaterals from history and mental status examination.

You describe the suspected diagnosis of MCI to the patient and his daughter. You let them know that while MCI identifies individuals with an increased risk

TABLE 6.3 Clinical insights for differentiating between normal aging, MCI, and MNCD

Neurocognitive domain	Description	Questions for patient and caregiver(s)	Diagnostic findings
Complex attention	Ability to focus on and carry out routine tasks or competing tasks in an appropriate amount of time	"When doing simple tasks with multiple distractions (e.g., TV, background conversations, music playing), how do you/the person respond?"	Normal aging: general slowing MCI: needs double-checking in routine tasks, slowing with simultaneous activities MNCD: unable to do simultaneous tasks unless simplified
Executive function	Multitasking or multistage actions	"When planning multistage tasks (e.g., paying bills, planning a visit to a friend), how do you/the person carry them out?" "Do you have any concerns about your/the person's driving?"	Normal aging: general slowing, insightful mistakes MCI: increased difficulty, fatigue; greater effort required MNCD: relies on others to plan tasks, can focus only on one task at a time. Insight and judgment are compromised.
Learning and memory	Remembering conversations; recalling recently introduced names, events, places	"During conversations, do you find yourself/the person repeating parts of conversations multiple times?"	Normal aging: forgetting names of familiar persons or where items were placed MCI: may repeat questions; needs reminders at times; more frequent memory lapses MNCD: frequent reminders in orienting to task at hand; declining short-term memory with increasing confabulations

Domain	Skill/Function	Question	Description
Language	Word-finding; grammar	"How do you/the person engage in routine conversations (e.g., telephone/dinner table)?"	Normal aging: not usually affected; subjective word-finding difficulty without substitutions MCI: socially noticeable word-finding difficulty MNCD: often substitutes general for specific terms; prefers general pronouns to names; may struggle to understand verbal requests (aphasia)
Perceptual-motor cognition	Tool-based tasks; navigating familiar environments	"How do you/the person go about doing known familiar tasks like using appliances or other household objects?"	Normal aging: not usually affected MCI: decreased use or more difficulty with using familiar household items or appliances MNCD: significant difficulties (apraxia)
Social cognition	Recognizing social cues and responding with appropriate behaviors and emotions	"How do you/the person behave in public around others and at social gatherings?"	Normal aging: not usually affected MCI: subtle episodes of discomfort, withdrawal, or faux pas in social settings; reduced ability to interpret facial expressions MNCD: progressive discomfort, disinterest, apathy, or social withdrawal; inappropriate or disinhibited responses or behaviors in social settings

of developing dementia, the outcome of an individual patient is not absolutely determined by the diagnosis. The daughter asks whether there are genetic factors that can clarify her father's likely diagnosis and course.

Unlike gene testing for mutations to predict rare familial early-onset dementia, predictive gene testing of the apolipoprotein E4 allele for late-onset Alzheimer's dementia is not recommended, as it does not improve the sensitivity and specificity of diagnosis, nor alter treatment strategies. It is best to explain that it is a susceptibility gene, meaning that a patient may carry high-risk alleles and not develop Alzheimer's dementia, or may develop Alzheimer's without them. *In this case, you suggest deferring the genetic testing.*

The clinical severity of MCI and the phenotype of the clinical syndrome are potential candidates for predicting progression. Additional neuropsychological testing may show evidence of depression and/or MCI with multiple domains of impairment (e.g., in executive dysfunction) in addition to memory. This phenotype is likely to progress more rapidly to a MNCD. It is important to remember that age, education, and culture influence a patient's performance on neuropsychological testing; hence, clinical judgment is always required when interpreting results.

Neuroimaging may enhance the predictive validity of progression to dementia. Hippocampal and entorhinal cortex atrophy has a small but detectable predictive utility over and above age and MCI in estimating risk of progression to probable Alzheimer's disease subtype of dementia. The presence of ischemic infarcts or hemosiderin deposits from prior intracerebral hemorrhages also increases the risk of Alzheimer's disease. Neuroimaging may also help with ruling out other causes of cognitive impairment.

The patient's mood and cognition improve from treatment of his depression and tapering of his benzodiazepine. He is then lost to follow-up. Three years later, he returns with progression of his memory deficits. He routinely forgets to pay his bills and avoids his usual social gatherings. He has had one episode of urinary incontinence, which he attributes to increased frequency. His medication list remains unchanged aside from the absence of the previously prescribed benzodiazepine. He remains independent in his self-care tasks but requires assistance in buying groceries and transportation. He has slowed down considerably and has had at least two falls in the last 2 months. He often repeats himself during conversations and uses general pronouns rather than names. He has "good days" and "bad days." He scores 21/30 on the MMSE, failing to reproduce the drawing of intersecting pentagons and missing several points on orientation and delayed recall. On examination, there are no signs of parkinsonism or focal neurologic deficits. He seems largely unconcerned about his deficits and minimizes their consequences.

DEMENTIA SUBTYPE AND STAGING

The patient now has an established MNCD (or dementia) and it is time to ascertain the subtype and stage. Key elements of history, examination, neuropsychological testing, and neuroimaging findings across the life history of the individual for the major subtypes of MNCDs are listed in Table 6.4. Staging can be accomplished by the use of tools like the Reisberg Functional Assessment Scale (FAST), which allows the caregiver to relate to functional stages of the illness and help match the patient's current functioning with the stage described.

The clinical diagnostic frame of mild MNCD of mixed subtype (Alzheimer's disease and vascular dementia) in this 69-year-old lawyer sets the stage for you to now discuss advance directives, independence and safety planning (e.g., driving, kitchen hazards), and implementing both pharmacologic and nonpharmacologic strategies.

KEY POINTS TO REMEMBER

- There is no single definitive diagnostic test or marker for neurocognitive disorders. Assessment requires clinicians to synthesize information from multiple data sources and assessments.
- Making a diagnosis involves initially establishing the extent and nature of cognitive deficits using clinical assessment and cognitive screening or neuropsychological testing.
- This information, combined with laboratory tests and neuroimaging, can help identify the MNCD subtype and track longitudinal progression of symptoms.

TABLE 6.4 Clinical insights for differential diagnosis of subtype of dementia

History and physical examination	Cognitive testing	Neuroimaging	Dementia subtype
Insidious onset of gradually progressive short-term memory deficits. Impairment in language, social graces, motor function (e.g., parkinsonism) occur later on. *On exam*: normal gait, short-term memory deficits, frontal release signs (advanced).	Impaired orientation, delayed recall, and executive function are the most prominent deficits.	Hippocampal and entorhinal cortex atrophy	Alzheimer's disease
Stepwise progression in cognitive impairment following vascular cerebral insults, vascular risk factors. *On exam*: stepwise progression of executive function deficits, pseudobulbar affect, apathy, slowing of gait, neuroanatomic -specific aphasias and motor deficits.	Verbal learning and recall less severe, prominent deficits in Trail Making. Deficits are associated with geographic infarcts.	Multiple strokes and/ or subcortical white matter lesions	Vascular dementia
Insidious onset, gradual progression of impairment in social graces, behaviors, or language. May be associated with parkinsonism or symptoms of motor neuron disease, compulsive or ritualistic behaviors. *On exam*: loss of object knowledge, with impoverished content, semantic and paraphasic errors, lack of empathy, frontal release signs.	Relatively preserved memory and visuospatial components. Prominent deficits in trail making, language, backward digit span.	Anterior cingulate, orbitofrontal, insular, and dorsolateral prefrontal atrophy, caudate and putamen involvement; or bilateral frontal lobe atrophy	Frontotemporal dementia

Clinical features	Cognitive findings	Imaging	Diagnosis
Insidious onset of visuospatial impairment (e.g., getting lost, difficult with arts and crafts or woodworking), hallucinations, history of rapid eye movement (REM) sleep behavior problems ("acting out dreams," sleepwalking), parkinsonism, fluctuating levels of alertness. Close onset of parkinsonism and cognitive impairment (within 12–18 months). *On exam:* parkinsonian features, antipsychotic hypersensitivity, marked fluctuations in cognitions and psychomotor functions.	Prominent visuospatial (clock drawing, intersecting pentagons) and attention deficits, milder deficits in confrontational naming. Impaired delayed free recall with preserved delayed recall with categorical cues (e.g., patient cannot recall the word "apple" spontaneously, but does so when the cue "fruit" is given).	Initially, normal; nonspecific atrophy that may vary with symptoms	Lewy body dementia
Insidious onset of executive functional and short-term memory impairment at least 4 years after the onset of motor symptoms of parkinsonism. Constipation and fatigue also noted. REM sleep behaviors and periodic limb movements may accompany. *On exam:* stooped posture, cogwheeling rigidity, akinesia, resting tremor. Normal extraocular movements.	Decreased executive function followed by short-term memory deficits	No typical structural MRI findings	Parkinson's disease dementia

Further Reading

Ahmed RM, Paterson RW, Warren JD, Zetterberg H, O'Brien JT, Fox NC, Halliday GM, Schott JM. Biomarkers in dementia: Clinical utility and new directions. *J Neurol Neurosurg Psychiatry*. 2014;85(12):1426–1434.

American Psychiatric Association. (2013). *Diagnostic and Statistical Manual of Mental Disorders* (5th ed.). Author.

Lenin ED. *Neurotransmitter Interactions and Cognitive Function*. Birkhäuser Verlag; 2006.

Miller B, Boeve B. *Behavioral Neurology of Dementia*. Cambridge University Press; 2009.

Petersen R, Doody R, Kurz A, Mohs R, Morris J, Rabins P, Ritchie K, Rossor M, Thal L, Winblad B. Current concepts in mild cognitive impairment. *Arch Neurol*. 2001;58:1985–1992.

Neurocognitive Disorders

7 Am I losing my mind?

Angela M. Kristan and
Elizabeth J. Santos

A 63-year-old woman comes to the clinic asking, "Am I losing my mind?" Since taking early retirement last year, she notes that she is having trouble concentrating on things, missing some appointments and forgetting a friend's birthday. She loved working as an elementary school teacher but retired early, believing that she could no longer keep up with the kids due to fatigue and diabetic neuropathy. She lies awake at night worrying about possibly having dementia like her mother did, and she does not want to be a burden to her family. Her husband reports that she is functioning very well at home and has no trouble with dressing or paying the bills. Her neurologic examination is normal, but she scores in the mildly impaired range on a cognitive screen.

What do you do now?

In this case, the patient is understandably concerned about noticeable cognitive changes and wonders if she is developing a dementia similar to what her mother had. To help her, the clinician must be able to distinguish between normal age-associated changes in cognition versus some objective form of neurocognitive decline such as mild cognitive impairment (MCI) or an actual dementia, now referred to as a major neurocognitive disorder (MNCD). With normal age, there are expected changes in cognitive function, including slower processing speed and access to working memory, which result in slower decision-making and executive function. At the same time, procedural and long-term memory are preserved with age, and there may even be improved vocabulary and general knowledge. Language comprehension is usually stable, with preserved understanding of written language, but there may be trouble understanding rapid speech. It is normal to have problems with selective attention and to be, as a result, more easily distracted and slower with switching sets or multitasking. One way of conceptualizing this is that "crystallized intelligence" or "wisdom" is preserved, but "fluid intelligence" is worse. For normal aging, one may notice that while it can take longer for older adults to carry out a task, they are still capable of completing it. One key factor to consider is that subjective reports of memory lapses and other cognitive changes may or may not represent actual objective changes; if they are present, they might be variable due to transient, reversible factors such as poor sleep, medications, or changes in mood.

For some individuals, objective changes go slightly beyond what we would expect for normal aging, based on normative scores, and this is referred to as MCI (or, alternatively, mild neurocognitive disorder). However, the objective impairment is less than that seen with MNCDs and does not significantly affect daily function. There are variable statistical cutoffs to define MCI on standardized testing, ranging from 1 to 1.5 standard deviations compared to age- and education-matched controls, depending on the test used. Common complaints in MCI include short-term memory lapses, word-finding problems, and getting lost in familiar places, but without the compromise in daily function and progressive decline seen in MNCDs.

In this case, the patient perceives cognitive changes related to concentration and forgetting things, but they do not affect her ability to care for herself or her family. She remains independent in terms of her activities of daily living (ADLs), such as managing her hygiene and grooming, and instrumental activities of daily living (IADLs), such as cooking, driving, and managing her finances. In addition, her husband is not concerned about her cognitive abilities. On the other hand, the patient does have a concerning family history of MNCDs in several family members. Putting everything together, she is best diagnosed with MCI. For a diagnosis of an MNCD to be made, she would need to have impairments in more than one cognitive domain that interfere with her ability to function independently.

SUBTYPES

There are four subtypes of MCI to note based on two criteria: amnestic versus non-amnestic and single domain versus multiple domains. The amnestic versus non-amnestic subtypes of MCI are diagnosed based on the presence or absence of memory loss (e.g., misplacing things or forgetting conversations). These are further subdivided by the number of neurocognitive domains that are impaired. Amnestic multidomain MCI is the most likely type to progress to dementia. In some studies, as many as 8 out of 10 patients with the amnestic type in multiple domains progress to dementia within 5 years. Thus, MCI represents a prodromal state of Alzheimer's disease (AD) or other forms of dementia in up to half of individuals, with the others either remaining the same or getting better. These findings show MCI to be an important early stage or window into potentially evolving neurocognitive conditions that warrant close assessment and follow-up.

RISK FACTORS AND CAUSES

The greatest risk factor for development of MCI is age. A meta-analysis conducted by the American Academy of Neurology found the estimated prevalence of MCI to be 8.4% of those 65 to 69, 10.1% of those age 70 to 74 years, 14.8% of those age 75 to 79, and 25.2% of those age 80 to 84. Other significant risk factors for development of MCI include:

- Lower educational level
- Vascular risk factors, including hypertension, midlife diabetes, and obesity
- History of stroke or heart disease
- Apolipoprotein E (*APOE*) epsilon 4 genotype
- Neuropsychiatric symptoms (e.g., agitation, apathy, depression, anxiety)

There are many potentially reversible causes of MCI. Many medications can interfere with cognitive function, whether they are prescribed or over-the-counter, especially ones that have anticholinergic or sedating properties. For example, many individuals who take over-the-counter sleep aids think they are innocuous, not realizing that an antihistamine such as diphenhydramine can affect memory and concentration. A good source to help identify potentially problematic medications in older patients is the American Geriatrics Society Beers Criteria.

Sleep problems such as chronic insomnia can certainly affect cognition. For this reason, it is prudent to consider obtaining a sleep study to evaluate for the quality of sleep and proper oxygenation and to rule out conditions such as obstructive sleep apnea (OSA) or restless legs syndrome. Improvement in sleep via proper sleep hygiene and use of a continuous positive airway pressure (CPAP) machine (in the case of OSA) can often result in corresponding improvements in attention and concentration.

Another common cause of MCI is psychiatric illness. Anxiety and mood disorders, in particular, can impair attention and concentration, leading, in turn, to memory and other cognitive lapses. Alcohol and other substance use disorders can impair cognition as well, both directly through acute intoxication and neurotoxic effects and indirectly through disruptions in sleep, nutrition, and medical stability as well as from medication interactions and falls and other injuries. Ideally, these potential causes and comorbidities of MCI will emerge as part of the history taking, but they also may be revealed through the use of standardized instruments such as the Beck Anxiety Index (BAI), the General Anxiety Disorder 7-item Scale (GAD-7), the Patient Health Questionnaire 9-item (PHQ-9), and the Center for Epidemiological Studies Depression Scale (CES-D), among others.

ASSESSMENT

The workup for MCI is complex, and collateral information is very important to the history taking. Collateral informants may not notice any problems and just suspect normal aging, or they may report only simple problems. If these problems are pointed out to the informant, they should agree that these problems do not affect daily function to be consistent with the diagnosis of MCI. Initial testing with a brief, validated cognitive screening assessment such as the Montreal Cognitive Assessment (MoCA), the St. Louis University Mental Status Exam (SLUMS), or the Mini–Mental State Exam (MMSE) should be done and followed at least annually. Scores on cognitive screening tools alone, however, cannot capture the range and myriad ways that one's mind works throughout the day to make both simple and sophisticated decisions. In fact, most individuals with MCI will score in normal to low-normal ranges on these instruments, and so more accurate diagnosis will require neuropsychological testing (see Chapter 4).

The physical and neurological exams should be conducted but are often unrevealing in MCI. A basic blood panel should include a complete blood count and basic metabolic panel, along with levels for vitamin B_{12}, vitamin D, thyroid stimulating hormone, and hemoglobin A1C. Brain imaging such as magnetic resonance imaging (MRI) is more sensitive than computed tomography (CT) scanning to assess patterns of atrophy, but the results will neither confirm nor rule out an MCI diagnosis. There is no clear role for any other imaging studies or electroencephalography (EEG) to diagnose MCI itself, although biomarker studies for AD, including both functional MRI and amyloid-based positron emission tomography (PET) scans, may determine the presence of MCI as an early-onset stage of AD.

TREATMENT

Once a diagnosis of MCI is made, it is critical to follow the patient clinically and to use consistent neuropsychological tests on at least an annual basis to determine any changes. Given the heterogeneity of MCI, there are no specific treatments recommended other than addressing underlying causes or exacerbating factors, minimizing medical and psychiatric comorbidities, and adopting a brain-healthy lifestyle. Such a lifestyle includes regular physical exercise, a healthy diet full of fruits and vegetables (with the best models being the Mediterranean, MIND, and DASH diets), regular socialization, regulation of blood pressure and glucose levels, adequate sleep, stress reduction, and brain-stimulating activities. Alcohol use should be limited to no more than one standard drink daily of wine, beer, or other spirits. Cognitive training exercises may be beneficial, with a focus on learning new skills and doing varied activities to challenge different parts of the brain.

No medications for MCI have been approved by the U.S. Food and Drug Administration (FDA), and the cognitive-enhancing medications used to treat AD and other MNCDs have not been shown to be effective. There are myriad "brain tonics" and other supplements on the market that tout memory improvement, but none has been shown to treat MCI, and few if any have any form of randomized controlled trials to even support their role with memory and learning. Nonetheless, many individuals indulge in these products and other substances, such as CBD oil, hoping for benefits that have never been proven scientifically.

Since there is a possibility that MCI may progress to dementia, future planning is important to consider while the patient has the ability to make complex decisions. Health care proxies, advance directives, and powers of attorney should be discussed with family and friends so that the patient's wishes are well known to everyone.

The patient describes anxiety due to her worries about having dementia like her mother did. She also feels depressed, and her Geriatric Depression Scale (GDS) score indicates a moderate level of depression. Since retiring from teaching, she has been less active and less connected to her closest friends, who are all teachers. When she does see her friends, she feels more disconnected as they talk about their work and school, and she has slowly withdrawn from contact with them. Treatment of her depression and anxiety should avoid benzodiazepines or antidepressants with any anticholinergic properties. Psychotherapy may help her to cope with her anxiety about possibly having dementia like her mother and to reconnect with friends despite her new role as a retired teacher. A brain-healthy lifestyle with a focus on physical exercise will enhance her well-being, improve brain blood flow and oxygenation, and improve her general physical and mental health. Hopefully, her MCI will not progress and may even improve over time.

- MCI represents a syndrome of objective cognitive change without significant functional impairment.
- Subjective memory complaints need to be evaluated with objective measures and correlated with functional abilities.
- Look for reversible, treatable conditions like sleep disorders, medication or substance effects, mood and anxiety disorders, or medical and neurologic conditions.
- There is no established treatment for MCI, but patients should be followed on a regular basis and prescribed a brain-healthy lifestyle.

Further Reading

Croke L. Beers criteria for inappropriate medication use in older patients: An update from the AGS. *Am Fam Physician*. 2020;101(1):56–57.

Kimchi EZ, Lyketsos CG. Dementia and mild neurocognitive disorders. In: Steffens DC, Blazer DG, Thakur ME, eds. *American Psychiatric Publishing Textbook of Geriatric Psychiatry* (5th ed.). American Psychiatric Publishing; 2015:177–242.

Langa KM, Levine DA. The diagnosis and management of mild cognitive impairment: A clinical review. *JAMA*. 2014;312(23):2551–2561.

Petersen RC, Lopez O, Armstrong MJ, et al. Practice guideline update summary: Mild cognitive impairment: Report of the Guideline Development, Dissemination, and Implementation Subcommittee of the American Academy of Neurology. *Neurology*. 2018;90(3):126–135.

8 I can't remember what just happened

Michael Li and Erica C. Garcia-Pittman

The patient is a 71-year-old man who was referred to a psychiatric clinic for memory problems. For the past year he has been forgetting conversations, misplacing items around the house, having difficulty managing emails, and has gotten lost a few times while driving. At the appointment, the patient was pleasant and spoke fluently, but had some difficulty finding the right words. He frequently asked to have questions repeated, but became slightly irritated when he needed prompting to respond. The evaluation revealed a likely diagnosis of Alzheimer's disease (AD), and the patient and his wife want to know his treatment options.

What do you do now?

AD is a neurodegenerative disorder that primarily affects older adults. It is the most common cause of dementia, and in the United States alone there are an estimated 5.6 million people age 65 and older who are living with this disease. With older age being the main risk factor, the sheer number of individuals with AD will increase significantly as the size of the U.S. population age 65 and older is set to increase from 55 million in 2019 to 88 million by 2050. Despite the urgency to help these individuals, only a limited number of treatment options have been approved by the U.S. Food and Drug Administration (FDA), and none of the available treatments reverse or stop the progression of AD. Thus, clinicians are faced with the challenge of selecting the type and timing of available interventions throughout the course of illness.

TREATMENT OF EARLY-STAGE, MILD AD

The patient's history indicates he is in an early and mild stage of AD, given his cognitive impairment primarily in the domains of learning, memory, and executive functioning coupled with generally independent functioning and needing only minor assistance in several areas. Common symptoms of early-stage AD include forgetting material that was just discussed, repeating oneself often, struggling with vocabulary and new names, misplacing objects more frequently, and having some difficulty with executive function, such as managing finances and cooking.

At this stage of illness, it would be appropriate to start patients on an acetylcholinesterase inhibitor (AChEI). Like the medication class name implies, AChEIs work by inhibiting the breakdown of acetylcholine in neural synapses, thus increasing the amount of this key neurotransmitter that is available for memory and learning. Most clinical studies of AChEIs examined patients in the mild to moderate stages of AD, and have shown measurable improvement of global functioning within the first year of treatment in memory, language, and praxis domains. Several studies have also suggested that AChEIs may blunt the prevalence of agitated behaviors and improve apathy.

Guidelines suggest that clinicians attempt at least a 6-month trial of a single AChEI and assess for clinical response, keeping in mind that even though AChEIs may provide benefit over 5 years or more, this does not represent any known pathologic slowing of the disease process itself. As a result, long-term evidence indicates that clinical improvement wanes over time, likely due to declining pools of acetylcholine-producing cells, and that patients will inevitably progress into a more severe stage of AD. While this may be a disheartening reality, blunting or even modestly improving the patient's symptoms can improve the quality of life for both patients and their caregivers, save on social and financial resources, and delay the time to long-term care placement. The current AChEIs approved by the FDA for mild and moderate stages of AD are listed in Table 8.1, with their respective preparations and dosing strategies.

Selecting the appropriate AChEI and formulation may be dependent on a patient's ability to tolerate medication side effects. The most common side effects include gastrointestinal issues (e.g., nausea, vomiting, loss of appetite, indigestion, weight loss, diarrhea), vivid dreams or nightmares, and the potential for increased pulmonary secretions and slowed heart rate, especially in individuals with preexisting vulnerabilities to either issue. It would be prudent to rule out any active heart conduction defects before initiating an AChEI due to the risk of bradyarrhythmia. Peripheral cholinergic side effects are usually dose-related and may resolve with time, dose reduction, or taking the medication with meals. Studies have suggested that donepezil has a lower risk of inducing gastrointestinal symptoms, so clinicians may consider switching a patient to this medication if the patient cannot tolerate either rivastigmine or galantamine. Patients taking oral rivastigmine may also consider switching to the patch or taking smaller doses more frequently throughout the day to mitigate gastrointestinal symptoms. Weight loss can also occur with AChEIs and may be complicated by anosmia and appetite loss due to AD itself. Therefore, it would be appropriate to consult a nutritionist, regularly monitor body mass index (BMI), and encourage caregivers to cook with enhanced flavors that may stimulate appetite. Nightmares may be a significant complaint in patients taking donepezil, as they can be both emotionally and behaviorally disruptive. Encouraging patients to take the medication earlier in the morning may improve these nocturnal disturbances.

In addition to cognitive-enhancing medication in early stages of AD, there are several nonpharmacologic approaches to be considered. Cognitive rehabilitation can include structured socialization (e.g., groups or clubs that do activities together), therapeutic activities (e.g., music, pet, and art

TABLE 8.1 AChEls for treating AD

Medication	Starting dose	Therapeutic dose	Titration strategy
Donepezil	Oral: 5 mg daily	Oral: 10 mg daily for mild-to moderate-stage AD Oral: 23 mg daily for severe stage	After 4–6 weeks of starting dose, may increase to 10 mg/day if minimal clinical improvement is seen. If patient tolerates treatment for ≥3 months but has symptoms of the severe stage, consider increasing dose to 23 mg/day
Galantamine	Oral IR: 4 mg twice a day with food Oral ER: 8 mg daily with food	Oral IR: 8–12 mg twice a day with food Oral ER: 16 or 24 mg daily with food	IR: May increase total daily dose by 8 mg (split into twice-a-day dosing schedule) every 4 weeks depending on tolerability and clinical improvement ER: May increase daily dose by 8 mg every 4 weeks depending on tolerability and clinical improvement
Rivastigmine	Oral: 1.5 mg twice a day with food Patch: 4.6 mg/24hours with food	Oral: 6 mg twice a day with food Patch: 9.5 to 13.3 mg/24 hours with food	Oral: May increase total daily dose by 3 mg (split into twice-a-day dosing schedule) every 2 weeks depending on tolerability Patch: May increase dose every 4 weeks to 9.5 mg/24 hours and 13.3 mg/24 hours, depending on tolerability and symptom severity

IR = immediate release; ER = extended release

therapy), and the use of computerized games to help patients maintain a good quality of life, enhance cognitive skills and compensate for specific areas of impairment, and improve mood and behavior. Some evidence supports the benefits of these varied approaches, although most studies vary in quality and consistency of effect. Several randomized controlled trials of AD patients participating in physical exercise regimens, even as simple as walking, have demonstrated improved memory and other cognitive skills; less anxiety, agitation, and depression; improved sleep and appetite; enhanced daily function; and decreased rates of falls and injury. These benefits are related to improved brain blood flow and release of neural growth factors and endogenous endorphins, as well as improved muscle tone, strength coordination, and balance. Occupational therapy can help patients and caregivers optimize basic perceptual motor skills, while speech therapy can improve language-processing skills and overall communication. Finally, there are several psychotherapeutic approaches, including problem-solving therapy, that can improve coping skills and reduce anxiety and depression. These approaches may be best administered by trained specialists. While digital tools such as apps have been developed for these indications, there is limited evidence to support their efficacy, and issues of data privacy and security must be considered.

TREATMENT OF MIDDLE- TO LATE-STAGE, MODERATE TO SEVERE AD

As individuals with AD progress into middle stages with moderate impairment in short-term memory and other cognitive skills, they require more assistance with both basic activities of daily living (ADLs; e.g., bathing, dressing, grooming, eating, ambulating, managing continence and toileting) and instrumental ADLs (personal transportation, shopping, preparing meals, housecleaning, managing medications, managing finances, and communicating with others by phone or mail). Individuals with more advanced or severe impairment in cognitive and functional skills have increasing difficulty communicating with others verbally and nonverbally and maintaining personal safety, and require increasing and eventually near-total supervision and assistance. In terminal stages, individuals lose the ability to talk, walk, manage continence, and eventually swallow.

The patient returned to the clinic regularly after initiating treatment with donepezil, and both he and his family reported modest improvement in his attention and memory once he started on the therapeutic dose of 10 mg daily. However, as his symptoms progressed into a more moderate stage of impairment, his short-term memory and other cognitive skills noticeably worsened, and he needed more supervision and help with his daily schedule and all transportation. At this point, it wasn't clear to what extent the medication was effective. He was taking donepezil which, like all other AChEIs, is indicated for mild to moderate AD. Unlike the others, however, donepezil is also indicated for severe AD. At this point it would make sense to attempt to increase the dose to the highest therapeutic level, which would be the slow-release 23-mg dose. Similarly, it would be appropriate to consider increasing a patient's therapeutic dose of galantamine from 16 mg (8 mg twice daily [for the immediate-release form] or 16 mg [for the extended-release form]) to 24 mg, or rivastigmine from the 9.5-mg/day patch to the 13.3-mg/day patch. Not all patients will tolerate these increases, however, and patients need to be monitored very carefully for emergent side effects such as gastrointestinal distress. As the patient progresses into a severe stage of illness, these higher dosing levels could be maintained.

There is another pharmacologic option for individuals at this point: memantine, a low-affinity NMDA (glutamate) receptor antagonist that has FDA approval for moderate to severe stages of AD. It regulates the activity of glutamate, which is a neurotransmitter involved in information processing and retrieval. High levels of glutamate stimulation may induce neuronal death, so memantine reduces the neurotoxic potential without interfering with glutamate's physiologic role. The primary evidence for NMDA antagonists is for moderate to severe stages of AD, where they showed small but clinically appreciable benefits on cognition and daily functioning, with modest risk reduction of patients developing agitation. It is important to note that several studies provide conflicting evidence where mild confusion and agitation developed in a few patients shortly after memantine was started. NMDA hypofunction within the limbic system has been deemed an underlying cause of psychosis, so it is possible that memantine may induce psychotic symptoms in a similar fashion to other glutamate receptor antagonists (e.g., phencyclidine, amantadine). However, this behavioral disturbance generally has an acute onset, occurring shortly after initiating memantine or increasing the dose (i.e., 1 week), and can be resolved by discontinuing the medication. It would be prudent for clinicians to clarify whether a patient has ever had a history of agitation with other cognitive-enhancing medications, as this could be a risk factor for memantine-induced agitation. Other potential side effects include constipation, headache, and hypertension. Table 8.2 provides information on memantine dosing.

TABLE 8.2   Dosing for memantine in treating AD

Dose	Titration strategy
Immediate release (oral): Start 5 mg daily; maximum 10 mg twice a day	Immediate release: Wait at least 1 week before increasing daily dose by 5 mg. Daily total doses >5 mg should be split into twice-a-day dosing
Extended release (oral): Start 7 mg daily; maximum 28 mg daily	Extended release: Wait at least 1 week before increasing daily dose by 7 mg until maximal dose is reached

Combination therapy with the cholinergic transmission enhancement of an AChEI and the prevention of neuronal degeneration by memantine is currently the standard of care in moderate to severe stages of AD. This is supported by a comprehensive study that followed patients over a 30-month period and found that combination therapy with memantine and an AChEI was superior in blunting cognitive and functional symptoms when compared to treatment with an AChEI alone or no treatment at all. Other research found a consistent benefit across cognitive, behavioral, and functional domains with combination therapy. In 2014 the FDA approved a fixed-dose oral combination formulation of memantine and donepezil for moderate to severe stages of AD. Clinicians may consider this formulation to reduce pill burden and facilitate ease of ingestion as patients may sprinkle the capsule onto food, though its clinical benefits remain similar to the generic combination.

OTHER TREATMENTS

The patient and his family initially noticed modest improvement and over time less decline in cognition and function on combination therapy. With time, however, the progressive decline into a more severe stage of AD prompted the family to ask about additional treatments.

At this stage, all of the nonpharmacologic strategies mentioned earlier in the chapter are relevant as long as they can be adapted to the patient's extant strengths (such as sensory abilities) and limitations. There is often more apathy along with behavioral changes and physical limitations that can offset any stability of functioning achieved during moderate stages. There has been research into nutritional approaches such as caprylic acid and coconut oil, which are theorized to be neuroprotective by providing an alternative energy source of ketone bodies to a brain that has lost the ability to metabolize glucose properly. Currently there is no evidence that supports any appreciable benefit from these or other supplements (e.g., coral calcium, ginkgo biloba, coenzyme Q10) in treating AD. Omega-3 fatty acids might have potential benefits for dementia in the context of reducing overall cardiovascular risk, but there is insufficient evidence to recommend this in the treatment or prevention of AD. Ginkgo biloba, which is thought to have anti-inflammatory and antioxidant properties that are neuroprotective, was found to be no better than placebo in preventing or treating AD in a large, multicenter phase 3 clinical trial.

The limitations of current treatments highlight the need to develop new strategies that actually modify the course of disease rather than simply improving symptoms. Of greatest interest is the use of immunotherapy using anti-amyloid or anti-tau antibodies to help mobilize extracellular amyloid plaques and intracellular tau tangles in the brain. Clinical studies have shown the ability of several anti-amyloid monoclonal antibodies (e.g., crenezumab, gantenerumab, aducanumab, donanemab) to mobilize a significant amount of plaque in the brain, but with variable degrees of symptomatic slowing. It is possible that one or more of these treatments will achieve FDA approval in the near future. Immunotherapy via active vaccination against Aβ-complexes has either failed to achieve efficacy or caused adverse events (e.g., meningoencephalitis) in early trials. Agents that target tau neurofibrillary tangles (e.g., paclitaxel, epothilone) are currently undergoing early trials but are limited by toxic side effects or lack of efficacy. Other strategies that inhibit the interaction between Aβ and ApoE either by modulating ApoE gene expression through small-peptide fragments have observed reduced Aβ accumulation, improved memory deficits, and reduced levels of brain-soluble tau aggregates in AD transgenic mouse models. Overall, more evidence for these novel treatments is needed before they can be recommended for clinical use.

- Treatment with an AChEI provides benefit in improving or blunting the cognitive and functional symptoms of patients with AD with mild to moderate impairment.
- Combination treatment with memantine and an AChEI is the standard of care with moderate to severe symptoms of AD, and may provide further benefit in blunting functional decline and behavioral disturbances and delaying long-term care placement.
- Nonpharmacologic strategies are important to improve quality of life and overall cognitive and functional engagement in all stages of AD.
- Novel experimental treatments show early signs of promise, but more clinical trials are needed to guide recommendations.

Further Reading

Alzheimer's Association. 2021 Alzheimer's Disease Facts and Figures. https://www.alz.org/media/Documents/alzheimers-facts-and-figures.pdf

Atri A, Shaughnessy LW, Locascio JJ, Growdon JH. Long-term course and effectiveness of combination therapy in Alzheimer disease. *Alzheimer Dis Assoc Disord.* 2008;22(3):209–221.

Cummings J, Ritter A, Zhong K. Clinical trials for disease-modifying therapies in Alzheimer's disease: A primer, lessons learned, and a blueprint for the future. *J Alzheimers Dis.* 2018;64(S1):S3–S22.

Long JM, Holtzman DM. Alzheimer disease: An update on pathobiology and treatment strategies. *Cell.* 2019;179(2):312–339.

9 He became a different person practically overnight

Matthew E. Kern, Jessica Stovall, and Prasad R. Padala

A 76-year-old African American man is brought in by his adult daughter because of a concern about his memory and behaviors that occurred "practically overnight" about a year ago. She reports that he has difficulty finding the right words when they speak on the phone, and has recently forgotten entire conversations. He was a "go-getter" in the past but has been less interested in golf, which used to be his passion. She has begun to help pay his bills and prepare meals for him since he was struggling with both tasks. After he got lost while driving one day, she brought him for an evaluation. His medical history includes hyperlipidemia, hypertension, diabetes, and coronary artery disease. He scored 21 out of 30 on the Montreal Cognitive Assessment (MoCA) with most deficits in visual-spatial/executive, naming, attention, and abstraction.

What do you do now?

Vascular dementia (VaD) is the second most common cause of dementia: It accounts for 14% to 16% of all cases among older adults. It is seen at higher rates among African Americans and those of Asian descent compared to Caucasians. Based on the area of vascular pathology and resulting clinical manifestations, VaD is broadly classified into cortical and subcortical dementias, with the latter representing subtypes such as Binswanger's disease, caused by atherosclerosis of arteries feeding subcortical white matter and structures such as the thalamus and basal ganglia. Diagnostic criteria from the National Institute of Neurological Disorders and Stroke (NINDS) require a person to show a significant decline in memory and other cognitive abilities that cause impaired functioning, combined with evidence of cerebrovascular disease on neuroimaging. Detecting these criteria requires a thorough clinical evaluation (including a detailed patient history and physical examination) along with magnetic resonance imaging (MRI) or computed tomography (CT) scanning of the brain.

DIAGNOSIS

There are several key factors in the diagnostic work-up that point toward a diagnosis of VaD. A patient's history is often notable for a rather sudden onset of symptoms, the presence of multiple vascular risk factors, and sometimes the temporal association of cognitive deficits with vascular events. Physical examination may show focal neurologic deficits that reflect underlying damage to specific regions of the brain, such as aphasia and right-sided hemiparesis from left-sided temporal and parietal lobe strokes, or slowed and unsteady gait from subcortical and/or cerebellar stroke. Neuropsychological testing may show prominent deficits in executive function and complex attention that reflect damage to subcortical regions that connect with frontal lobe neural circuits. There is no specific test or lab value reflective of VaD, but clinicians should be mindful of abnormalities that increase the risk of cerebrovascular damage, including high blood pressure, hyperlipidemia, and elevated glucose and hemoglobin A1C levels. Other labs such as a comprehensive metabolic panel, thyroid function, folate, vitamin B_{12}, complete blood count, and an erythrocyte sedimentation rate are important but not diagnostic.

Neuroimaging is perhaps the most important test in the clinical work-up of a patient suspected of having VaD. The radiologic findings should meet the minimum standards of the NINDS criteria for both severity and topography to be considered evidence of probable VaD. Keep in mind that VaD is a heterogenous entity, including both large- and small-vessel disease, and involving gray and/or white matter. Small-vessel disease is the more common pathology and often presents as diffuse white matter changes and multiple lacunar infarcts. Large-vessel disease manifests as one or more strategic infarcts. The most important parameters underlying the clinical manifestations of VaD are the locations of the lesions, volume of destroyed tissue, multiplicity, and bilateral occurrence. Confluent white matter lesions need to involve at least 25% of the total white matter to reach the diagnosis of VaD. Lacunar infarcts need to involve multiple basal ganglia and the frontal white matter, and thalamic lesions need to be bi-lateral. Likewise, large-vessel disease needs to include at least one of the following territories: bilateral cerebral artery, paramedian thalamic, inferior medial temporal lobe, parieto-temporal and temporo-occipital association areas and angular gyrus, superior frontal and parietal watershed areas in the dominant hemisphere.

Patients with suspected VaD should also be screened for depression and apathy, which are common comorbidities. Vascular depression, a concept described and popularized by Alexopoulos and colleagues, is highly comorbid in patients with VaD due to the accompanying white matter changes and prominent executive dysfunction. The presence of executive dysfunction associated with VaD is predictive of depressive states that are less responsive to treatment. Apathy is a disorder of behavioral initiation that manifests as slowed but not necessarily impaired cognition, constricted emotional expression but not depression, and failure to initiate activities of daily living. Although there is overlap with depressive symptoms, mounting evidence shows apathy as a distinct entity that lacks dysphoria, suicidal ideation, self-criticism, and hopelessness.

The patient and his daughter returned for a follow-up visit 6 months after the initial evaluation. The mental status exam indicated that his mood was generally stable with some mild grief, along with continued apathy. Throughout the interview he would lose his attention when not addressed directly. He was able to remember two of five objects, but became frustrated with spelling, calculation, and animal naming tasks. He was near-oriented to date, but incorrectly identified the city he was in. Overall, his cognition did not show significant change from his baseline. There were no new physical findings or falls reported. The prior lab work was within normal limits, and his head CT showed moderate volume loss and evidence of ischemic changes with prominent changes in the left supplementary motor area. His occupational therapy assessment suggested that he not live independently, and he failed a driving test. His sleep study showed obstructive sleep apnea, though he has not been using his continuous positive airway pressure (CPAP) machine on a regular basis because he didn't understand how to wear the facemask properly.

The patient's clinical picture remains consistent with VaD and common associated comorbidities. The progression of VaD is highly variable. Unlike other types of dementia, it is difficult to predict the advancement of symptom burden because of the many factors that can trigger or mitigate further cerebrovascular compromise in so many different patterns. Sometimes, family members will observe an acute change, while other times the decline is quite subtle and small events, such as a lacunar infarct, will be missed entirely and not appreciated until there is an aggregation of damage. In many cases there can be improvement if there are no further cerebrovascular events or minimal progression of cerebrovascular disease, allowing time for the brain to recuperate to some extent.

MANAGEMENT

The management of VaD is multidisciplinary and comprises vascular risk management, counseling to optimize daily function and safety, and nonpharmacologic and pharmacologic management of cognitive and non-cognitive symptoms. An initial priority is to lower the patient's risk for more cerebrovascular events and damage. In this case, a good adage is "what's good for the heart is good for the brain," and so a brain-healthy lifestyle will include regular physical activity, a healthy diet, and aggressive identification and treatment of risk factors such as hyperlipidemia, diabetes, and hypertension. Nutritional approaches also play a prominent role, particularly a combination of a Mediterranean diet with the Dietary Approaches to Stop Hypertension (DASH) diet known as the MIND Diet, which has shown both dementia risk reduction and a potentially positive effect on memory. The MIND Diet emphasizes whole grains, healthier fats (e.g., olive oil), nuts, legumes, poultry, lots of fruits and vegetables, and even a single glass of wine, and de-emphasizes red meat, carbohydrates, and processed foods. A brain-healthy lifestyle also promotes good sleep, especially since obstructive sleep apnea is a common comorbidity in this population that is important to treat. The use of CPAP confers not only a cognitive benefit through improved sleep quality but also reduces the patient's risk of cardiovascular events.

Nonpharmacologic approaches to management should include regular brain-stimulating activities, such as structured computer games, art and music therapy, social activities, and physical exercise. The living environment should be adapted to specific cognitive deficits, such as putting up a large-print calendar, a list of important phone numbers near the telephone, and written reminder cards about taking medications or going to appointments. Attention to proper sleep hygiene can help reduce the impact of sleep disorders, improve brain alertness during the day, and lessen the use of sleeping pills, which often have anticholinergic side effects, including memory impairment.

The are several pharmacologic options for the management of symptoms in established VaD. The acetylcholinesterase inhibitors (AChEIs) donepezil, rivastigmine, and galantamine are approved by the U.S. Food and Drug Administration (FDA) for treating mild to moderate Alzheimer's disease (AD), but have also been used to treat VaD based on the belief that cholinergic deficits are common causes of cognitive impairment for both forms of dementia. Similarly, memantine has been used in VaD as an adjunct to AChEIs. There is some evidence to back up the efficacy of both classes of cognitive enhancers in VaD, with the same dosing strategies and side effect issues as with AD (see Chapter 8). It is important to educate families about the modest potential benefits of these medications, and to monitor closely for efficacy as well as side effects.

KEY POINTS TO REMEMBER

· VaD is suspected in patients with a significant cardiovascular history, cognitive decline associated with cerebrovascular

events, cardiovascular risk factors such as high blood pressure and diabetes, and neuroimaging findings of significant cerebrovascular injury.
- There are many variations of vascular dementia based on the location and degree of brain damage, with cortical and subcortical subtypes being one major distinction.
- Treatment should focus on reducing known risk factors in order to prevent or mitigate further cerebrovascular damage, and the use of both AChEIs and memantine as used to treat AD.
- Depression and apathy are relatively more common in VaD and should be routinely evaluated.

Further Reading

Padala PR, Padala KP, Lensing SY, Ramirez D, Monga V, Bopp MM, Roberson PK, Dennis RA, Petty F, Sullivan DH, Burke WJ. Methylphenidate for apathy in community-dwelling older veterans with mild Alzheimer's disease: A double-blind, randomized, placebo-controlled trial. *Am J Psychiatry.* 2018;175(2):159–168.

Porsteinsson AP, Drye LT, Pollock BG, Devanand DP, Frangakis C, Ismail Z, Marano C, Meinert CL, Mintzer JE, Munro CA, Pelton G, Rabins PV, Rosenberg PB, Schneider LS, Shade DM, Weintraub D, Yesavage J, Lyketsos CG; CitAD Research Group. Effect of citalopram on agitation in Alzheimer disease: The CitAD randomized clinical trial. *JAMA.* 2014;311(7):682–691.

Taylor WD, Aizenstein HJ, Alexopoulos GS. The vascular depression hypothesis: Mechanisms linking vascular disease with depression. *Mol Psychiatry.* 2013;18(9):963–974.

10 The man who mistook the trash for his dog

David Merril and Melita Petrossian

A 74-year-old retired attorney began experiencing deficits in short-term memory such as the inability to remember whether he had taken his medications. These cognitive deficits progressively worsened over several years, and he began to develop slowness of gait and other movements. He started having violent nightmares during which he would kick and punch into the air, prompting his wife to sleep in a separate bed to avoid injury. He reported visual hallucinations such as seeing small children walking around the house, or a nonexistent friend sitting at the end of his table. Some days he feels relatively clear, while other days he is more confused and psychotic. He saw a neurologist, who noted on exam that the patient had rigidity, bradykinesia, resting tremor, and postural instability. The doctor started him on levodopa with no motor improvement but increased psychosis.

What do you do now?

The combination of symptoms in this patient include features of Parkinson's disease (PD), psychosis, and cognitive dysfunction. Patients who present with cardinal features of parkinsonism are often suspected of having PD and treated as such; however, when standard medications for PD have insufficient effect and there are other telltale symptoms, the clinician should suspect dementia with Lewy bodies (DLB). Core features of DLB include the following:

- The presence of progressive cognitive impairment before the appearance of motor symptoms
- An unsatisfactory response to levodopa
- Prominent visual hallucinations
- Fluctuating symptoms (particularly transient changes in orientation and awareness)
- Sleep disturbances suggestive of rapid eye movement (REM) sleep behavior disorder (RBD)

The neuropsychological patterns observed in patients with DLB typically include executive dysfunction, delays in processing speed, and visuospatial deficits. Amnestic declines in DLB often result from difficulties in retrieval rather than deficits in encoding, whereas in AD, amnestic declines would typically involve encoding as well as retrieval. One challenge in differentiating DLB from dementia due to AD is the often equivocal nature of parkinsonism. For instance, slowed movement due to arthritic joints can mimic the appearance of bradykinesia; an inability to relax can suggest the appearance of rigidity; and a severe essential tremor with mixed action and rest tremor can be confused with the tremor seen in DLB. Psychotic symptoms are typically quite prominent early on, and medications used to treat them sometimes result in acute confusion.

Beyond the core clinical features of DLB, supportive features can be useful if identified but are not required for a clinical diagnosis. These include autonomic dysfunction (e.g., neurogenic orthostatic hypotension, urinary bladder dysfunction, constipation); transient, unexplained loss of consciousness or syncope; frequent falls; hyposmia or anosmia; and hypersomnia. While the hallucinations of DLB are typically visual, ranging from vague shapes to children, animals, or people, non-visual hallucinations can occur, including auditory and somatic hallucinations. Delusions (fixed false beliefs such as paranoia, delusions of reference, and misidentifications) can occur, but are not considered a core feature. Other common psychological symptoms include apathy, anxiety, and depression.

RBD refers to a sleep disturbance that primarily affects men over the age of 50, wherein a patient physically acts out dreams while asleep. During REM sleep, the body is normally paralyzed while the eyes move rapidly in different directions (hence "rapid eye movement" sleep). In RBD, the body is *not* paralyzed, and the dreamer may kick, punch, scream, or attempt to get out of bed. Typically, the dreams in RBD are violent in nature, but the dreamer is not the primary aggressor, meaning the patient is attempting to escape or fight off an attack on himself or a loved one. RBD is characterized by a loss of skeletal muscle atonia during REM sleep. REM sleep without atonia (RSWA) is denoted by increased phasic or tonic activity of the muscles, which can be diagnosed via sleep study (polysomnography [PSG]). RBD should be distinguished from sleep-related jerks, known as "myoclonus," and nightmares without dream enactment. RBD can precede the development of alpha-synucleinopathy by many years, and is a known harbinger for neurodegeneration. In fact, 70% to 90% of RBD patients who receive continued follow-up over 10 to 20 years are diagnosed with a neurodegenerative disease, such as idiopathic PD, DLB, multiple system atrophy, and/or, less commonly, Alzheimer's disease (AD).

Certain laboratory and imaging biomarkers can have a valuable role in elucidating an accurate diagnosis. When available, DaTscan (GE Healthcare), a dopamine transporter (DAT) single photon emission computed tomography (SPECT) imaging technique, or F-DOPA-PET, can detect deficits in presynaptic dopamine in the caudate and putamen—a biomarker of parkinsonism. Another diagnostic biomarker with a high degree of accuracy for Lewy bodies is iodine 131 metaiodobenzylguanidine (MIBG) myocardial scintigraphy. MIBG scintigraphy can reveal pathologically reduced myocardial MIBG uptake in both PD and DLB patients, and can function as another method of distinguishing between DLB and AD. Finally, PSG can be obtained to assess for REM sleep without atonia, a marker for RBD.

Idiopathic PD often progresses to dementia, typically beginning years after the onset of motor symptoms. As noted earlier, RBD is also common in patients with PD. Thus, distinguishing between PD dementia (PDD) and DLB can be very challenging. Many experts now characterize PDD and DLB as diseases existing on opposite ends of a single spectrum of Lewy body disease. For practical purposes, the primary feature differentiating PDD and DLB is the timing of the onset of dementia. In PDD, dementia typically begins years after the onset of parkinsonism, whereas in DLB, the cognitive symptoms begin either at the same time or years prior to the onset of movement symptoms. Furthermore, patients with DLB have a worse prognosis and a faster rate of disease progression compared to PD patients. The biomarkers discussed earlier are typically unable to differentiate reliably between DLB and PDD.

TREATMENT

Differentiating among PDD, AD, and DLB has prognostic and disease management implications. Medications such as levodopa and dopamine agonists, which are known to be beneficial for the motor symptoms of PD, tend to be less helpful for the motor symptoms of DLB; additionally, in patients with DLB, these drugs often have an increased rate of side effects, such as confusion and hallucinations. Patients with DLB are more likely to experience a paradoxical worsening of agitation when they are given antipsychotics, especially more potent dopamine receptor antagonists such as risperidone and haloperidol. Conversely, compared to patients with AD, those with DLB tend to experience more significant improvements in cognitive function with acetylcholinesterase inhibitors (AChEIs) such as donepezil, rivastigmine, and galantamine. While no medications are specifically approved by the U.S. Food and Drug Administration (FDA) for use in DLB, rivastigmine is approved for PDD, and the off-label use of AChEIs is well supported. In addition, data from several randomized controlled trials support the use of memantine for DLB.

Certain lifestyle measures, such as exercise, a Mediterranean diet, and sleep hygiene, have consistently been associated with improved cognitive outcomes in a broad range of neurodegenerative disorders, and thus are reasonable recommendations for patients and their families until further research has been conducted. Because many patients move impulsively and have retropulsion, they may benefit from physical and occupational therapy and appropriate measures to prevent falls, such as the use of a walker and the installation of grab bars in the shower and near the toilet.

Medications for motor parkinsonism such as levodopa can be considered with caution; it is important to recognize that DLB patients may experience a decreased response rate and more side effects than PD patients, especially confusion and hallucinations. Moreover, dopamine agonists and amantadine may be less effective than levodopa in DLB patients, and can cause or exacerbate hallucinations. Anticholinergics such as trihexyphenidyl should be avoided given the high risk of new or worsening confusion associated with their use in DLB. Interestingly, recent research has suggested the potential of AChEIs such as rivastigmine and donepezil in the management of the motor symptoms of PD, such as freezing of gait and falling.

Psychiatric issues such as agitation and psychosis should be managed primarily through the use of nonpharmacologic methods, which often requires caregiver training and education. Ideally, care partners should respond in a nonjudgmental, calm, and reassuring manner to the patient's described experience of a hallucination or delusion to reduce any associated anxiety and agitation. These approaches, as well as the avoidance of arguments regarding the patient's delusional beliefs, may reduce the frequency of behavioral outbursts. In some cases, the hallucinations may be mild and not bothersome to the patient, and thus can be managed conservatively. Rivastigmine has been shown to reduce the frequency of hallucinations and associated anxiety. Antipsychotics should be used carefully and in low doses given the higher frequency of side effects in patients with DLB. Although atypical antipsychotics such quetiapine are often prescribed for psychotic symptoms, there has been limited research to support its use. Pimavanserin is a serotonin 5-HT2A receptor inverse agonist that has FDA approval for the management of psychotic symptoms in PD, and was shown in one study of patients with DLB to reduce psychotic relapse compared to placebo. Mood and anxiety disorders in DLB can be treated with antidepressants such as selective serotonin reuptake inhibitors (SSRIs) and others.

Treatment of RBD should focus on the safety of the patient and bed partner. Because of the typically violent nature of their dreams, patients and their families should be advised to remove from the bedroom anything that could be used as a weapon, and firearms should be kept locked and unloaded. Some patients and families choose to apply soft padding to sharp corners on bedside tables, increase the use of pillows on the side of the patient and between the bed partners, and install bedrails to prevent the patient from jumping out of bed. Often, the patient's bed partner chooses to sleep in a separate room. The door of the bedroom should be kept closed if the bedroom is not on the first floor.

Pharmacologic treatment of RBD can be instituted if the behaviors are consistently threatening the patient's safety and/or quality of sleep. Melatonin is often a safe first-line medication in doses ranging from 3 to 15 mg, but there are limited data in non-DLB patients with RBD. One small randomized controlled trial of melatonin 3 mg demonstrated improvements in clinical and PSG measures in RBD, although most subjects had neither PD nor DLB. In another small randomized controlled trial in the treatment of RBD in individuals with PD, melatonin was no better than placebo. Clonazepam has also been used in the treatment of RBD, although the results of several studies have been inconsistent. Benzodiazepines such as clonazepam should be used with caution given the risk of exacerbating imbalance, fall risk, and confusion.

Several commonly prescribed drugs can cause or exacerbate DLB symptoms and must be used with extreme caution, including (1) anticholinergics, such as oxybutynin and diphenhydramine, which can cause acute confusion; (2) typical antipsychotics, such as haloperidol, which carry a high risk of worsening symptoms; and (3) dopamine-blocking antinausea medications such as metoclopramide and prochlorperazine, which can exacerbate motor symptoms of parkinsonism. Some patients with DLB also experience orthostatic hypotension, which can be exacerbated by alpha-blockers such as tamsulosin that are commonly prescribed for urinary symptoms of prostate hypertrophy. Dopamine agonists can worsen RBD and hallucinations, and amantadine and levodopa can exacerbate hallucinations and confusion. In general, individuals with DLB often show paradoxical reactions to many psychotropic medications, so dosing should always be conservative, with close monitoring.

The management of DLB requires a multidisciplinary approach to support the patient and caregivers. In addition to neurology, psychiatry, and primary care, the DLB team may include physical, occupational, and speech therapists, psychologists, social workers, case managers, and nurse specialists. Driving evaluations can be performed by occupational therapists, as issues of cognition, reaction timing, and/or visuospatial difficulties may preclude safe driving. The living situation can be assessed by case managers and nurse specialists to determine the optimal balance between independence and safety for the patient and loved ones. Because of the challenges of providing care to a patient with behavioral issues, caregiver self-care and respite are key. End-of-life care may include a consultation with palliative care specialists, the creation of advance directives for healthcare-related powers of attorney, and physician orders for life-sustaining treatment, to support the patient and family in dignified care that is commensurate with the patient's wishes.

The patient was gradually tapered off levodopa, and showed a mild improvement in daytime alertness without the worsening of motor symptoms. He was started on rivastigmine, which decreased the frequency and severity of hallucinations and mildly improved executive and short-term memory functioning. The patient was referred for physical and occupational therapy, and exercise was emphasized. He saw a stabilization of his motor symptoms and cognitive decline, and he experienced better day-to-day functioning for a short period of time. The family was grateful for the improved behaviors and quality of home life.

KEY POINTS TO REMEMBER

- In DLB, cognitive symptoms typically develop before or concurrent with parkinsonism, while in PDD, cognitive symptoms normally begin more than a year after the onset of movement symptoms.
- The core clinical features of DLB are dementia plus RBD, parkinsonism, visual hallucinations, and/or transient fluctuations in awareness.
- Antipsychotics, especially typical antipsychotics, should be avoided given the increased risk of mortality when used in patients with dementia and the higher frequency of side effects in patients with DLB.

Further Reading

Armstrong MJ, Alliance S, Corsentino P, DeKosky ST, Taylor A. Cause of death and end-of-life experiences in individuals with dementia with Lewy bodies. *J Am Geriatr Soc.* 2019;67(1):67–73.

Hansen D, Ling H, Lashley T, Holton JL, Warner TT. Review: Clinical, neuropathological and genetic features of Lewy body dementias. *Neuropathol Appl Neurobiol.* 2019;45(7):635–654.

Morrin H, Fang T, Servant D, Aarsland D, Rajkumar AP. Systematic review of the efficacy of non-pharmacological interventions in people with Lewy body dementia. *Int Psychogeriatr.* 2018;30(3):395–407.

Suddenly carefree and careless

Anil Vatsavayi

A 49-year-old business executive with no significant past medical or psychiatric history was evaluated for a 2-year history of progressive behavioral changes. His family history was notable for progressive psychiatric disorders in his father and paternal grandfather with onset in their 40s. The patient's psychiatric evaluation was remarkable for inappropriate and disorganized behaviors, hypomania, agitation, and mood lability. His neurologic examination was unremarkable. His wife described him becoming less sociable but more inappropriate. For example, he began making sexually inappropriate comments to women, and then started an extramarital affair and did not care if everyone knew. He was spending a lot of money buying and hoarding baseball equipment, and he started eating large amounts of ice cream and cake. Of note, the patient did not seem to understand nor care that his behaviors were affecting his family and friends.

What do you do now?

This case exemplifies that diagnosis in patients with late-onset neuropsychiatric disorders can be challenging due to overlapping symptomatology. The diagnosis appears to be an adult-onset mental illness or early-onset major neurocognitive disorder. The symptom complex with pronounced personality changes, disinhibition, loss of empathy, compulsive behaviors, and family history of late-onset progressive neuropsychiatric conditions makes a compelling case that this patient most likely has the behavioral variant of frontotemporal dementia (FTD). Given its heterogenous presentation, FTD is frequently misdiagnosed as a psychiatric disorder.

WHAT IS FTD?

FTD is a heterogenous neurodegenerative disorder characterized by progressive impairments in behavior, language, social cognition, and executive function. The clinical phenotypes of FTD are a behavioral variant (bvFTD) and a language variant referred to as primary progressive aphasia (PPA) with three subtypes: semantic variant PPA, nonfluent variant PPA, and logopenic variant PPA. Core clinical features are outlined in Table 11.1. The spectrum of FTD-like conditions includes corticobasal syndrome, progressive supranuclear palsy syndrome, and FTD motor neuron disease. Although considered a rare disease, FTD is the third most common form of dementia across all age groups, and the most common dementia in individuals less than age 60. The estimated lifetime risk of FTD is 1 in 742, with an incidence of 3.5 cases per 100,000 person-years in adults aged 45 to 64 years, and the prevalence is 15 to 22 per 100,000. There is no significant gender disparity. The median life expectancy is 7 to 8 years after symptom onset, with a variable rate of progression. Psychotic symptoms can occur in approximately 20% to 80% of FTD patients. Late-onset FTD often may be misdiagnosed as Alzheimer's disease (AD) or other major neurocognitive disorder.

In the fifth edition of the American Psychiatric Association's *Diagnostic and Statistical Manual of Mental Disorders* (DSM-5), diagnosis of bvFTD requires meeting criteria for a mild or major neurocognitive disorder including insidious onset and gradual progression combined with three or more behavioral symptoms and a prominent decline in social cognition

TABLE 11.1 FTD variants, clinical features, and affected brain regions

Phenotype	Clinical presentation	Affected brain regions
bvFTD	Emergence of abnormal behaviors, including: · Behavioral disinhibition · Loss of empathy · Apathy · Compulsive/perseverative behaviors · Hyperorality · Executive dysfunction	Atrophy in bilateral frontal lobes (esp. medial frontal lobes) and anterior temporal lobes
Semantic variant PPA	Impairments in semantic memory, including: · Word retrieval · Object naming (anomia) and recognition of its purpose or use (agnosia) · Single-word comprehension (especially for less familiar, less frequently used words) · Surface dyslexia (difficulty reading and writing words that do not have clear rules for pronunciation or spelling) · Speech production typically preserved	Atrophy in bilateral and asymmetric anterior, middle, and inferior temporal lobes, and ipsilateral orbitofrontal lobe
Nonfluent/ agrammatic variant PPA	Motor speech difficulties, including: · Slowed, effortful, nonfluent speech with speech sound errors, short phrases, frequent pauses and hesitancy · Agrammatic language production · Impaired comprehension of grammar and complex syntax	Atrophy in left hemisphere posterior fronto-insular, premotor, and anterior–superior temporal regions
Logopenic variant PPA	· Phonologic errors · Word-finding difficulties · Impaired sentence repetition	Atrophy in left hemisphere posterior temporal–parietal junction

and executive abilities, with relative sparing of learning, memory, and perceptual-motor function. The five behavioral symptoms are disinhibition; loss of sympathy or empathy; apathy or inertia; perseverative, stereotyped, or compulsive/ritualistic behaviors; and hyperorality/dietary changes. These impairments cannot be explained by other neurodegenerative processes, cerebrovascular disease, or other neurologic, psychiatric, or systemic disorders and are not substance-related. A diagnosis of *possible* bvFTD is made when it is based solely on clinical criteria; probable bvFTD can be diagnosed when there is either evidence of a causative genetic mutation from family history or genetic testing, or neuroimaging showing disproportionate frontal and temporal lobe involvement. The PPA variant of FTD involves semantic dysfunction. Its variants are described in Table 11.1 and the disorder is further classified as being with or without behavioral disturbances.

MAKING THE DIAGNOSIS

Current literature indicates that most FTD patients are initially assessed in general psychiatric settings, and about 50% receive a primary psychiatric diagnosis. Certain clinical features may suggest a neurodegenerative condition rather than a primary psychiatric disorder. These characteristics include new-onset personality change with psychiatric symptoms around age 40, progressive deterioration and atypical symptoms for a primary psychiatric disorder, no significant past psychiatric history, family history of early-onset dementia, new-onset seizures, and development of neurologic signs, including parkinsonism, dysarthria, apraxia, primitive reflexes, pseudobulbar affect, abnormal eye movements, and upper/lower motor neuron signs.

Given the wide-ranging and profound neuropsychiatric symptoms, especially in bvFTD, clinicians should rule out the multitude of psychiatric disorders exhibiting similar characteristics. For example, avolition, apathy, and poverty of speech seen in bvFTD may indicate negative symptoms in schizophrenia or major depressive disorder. Euphoria, irritability, and personality manifestations might suggest bipolar or personality disorder. Other common misdiagnosis includes early-onset AD, adult-onset attention-deficit/hyperactivity disorder (ADHD), obsessive–compulsive disorder, catatonia, and autism spectrum disorder. Also, the medical and public perception of dementia as an elderly medical condition, poor patient insight, and paucity of disease-specific biomarkers contribute to the misdiagnosis of bvFTD. Although less common, patients with a primary psychiatric disorder may be erroneously diagnosed with bvFTD in the setting of neuro-imaging misinterpretations or inaccurate history.

bvFTD can be diagnosed clinically through a comprehensive psychiatric interview, which includes a careful history of the illness, family history, mental status examination with a screening cognitive test, and a neurologic exam for signs of apraxia, parkinsonism, and motor neuron disease. The most distinct early symptoms of bvFTD are personality changes, disinhibition, loss of empathy, compulsive/perseverative behaviors, apathy, and dietary changes (Table 11.2). History should be obtained from both the patient and at least one knowledgeable informant and should involve exploring the time course, nature of symptoms, functional impairments, and cognitive decline. Patients often do not recognize many of the changes reported by collateral contacts due to their limited insight. A detailed family history of first- and second-degree relatives for psychiatric and neurologic disorders, especially a history of early-onset dementia, is an essential component of assessment. Late-onset psychiatric illness or unexplained institutionalization in a mental health facility should raise suspicion for familial bvFTD.

The evaluation should include routine laboratory testing to identify metabolic or reversible causes of neurocognitive impairment. In cases with a high degree of clinical suspicion, specialized evaluation for neurodegenerative diseases should be pursued aggressively. Persistent and progressive executive function and language impairments regardless of improvement in psychiatric symptoms may be suggestive of bvFTD rather than a psychiatric condition. Performance on standard screening tests may be within normal limits in early bvFTD; however, comprehensive testing may identify subtle deficits. Therefore, in patients presenting with progressive cognitive impairment in the setting of new onset of a psychiatric condition, neuropsychological testing can help identify the degree of executive dysfunction and signs of relative sparing of memory and visuospatial function. Keep in mind that social cognition deficits are among the earliest impairments in bvFTD but are inadequately detected by standard cognitive tests.

TABLE 11.2 **Behavioral and neuropsychiatric symptoms characteristic of bvFTD**

Symptom domains	Disinhibition	Personality changes	Compulsive behaviors	Dietary changes
Core features	Impaired impulse control, emotional/behavioral dysregulation, and inability to understand social/emotional cues - Impulsive, careless, rash actions - Socially inappropriate behaviors - Loss of embarrassment and sense of disgust - Loss of manners, etiquette	New, out-of-character behaviors - Loss of empathy and sympathy - Apathy and inertia - Deceased self-conscious emotions	Cognitive and behavioral rigidity - Simple repetitive movements - Complex, compulsive/ritualistic behaviors - Stereotypy of speech	Hyperorality - Altered food preferences - Oral exploration, consumption of inedible objects
Clinical scenarios	Invade physical/social space: Overly friendly, inappropriate touching of strangers/objects - Offensive jokes/comments - Profane language - Sexual remarks, advances - Childish behaviors - Poor personal hygiene - Reckless spending - Poor fiscal decisions	· Reduced interest in work, hobbies, social interaction, and hygiene · Emotional blunting · Diminished response to other people's needs/feelings, personal warmth, and interrelatedness	· Hoarding · Echolalia and perseverations · Simple stereotypies: humming, tapping, picking · Complex rituals: sequential actions, pacing, repetitive checking	· Increased consumption of sweets, alcohol, or cigarettes · Binge eating · Weight gain

- Work problems

- Alienation of family, friends

- New addictions

Legal problems due to new criminal behaviors: Theft, urination in public, careless driving (hit-and-run accidents), confrontational behaviors, altercations with strangers

Improper table manners: Eating with hands, licking plate, eating from other people's plates, picking up/eating food off the floor, searching trash for food

Neuroimaging plays an important role in the diagnosis of bvFTD and is indicated in late-onset mental illness with suspected bvFTD. Structural and functional neuroimaging can aid in the diagnosis by identifying patterns of atrophy, functional connectivity, and hypometabolism. A reasonable initial approach is structural imaging with computed tomography (CT) or magnetic resonance imaging (MRI), including the coronal and sagittal planes. Brain MRI permits a more accurate definition of boundaries between cerebrospinal fluid (CSF) and brain parenchyma and therefore provides a more sensitive evaluation of atrophy patterns. bvFTD is associated with predominant frontal and temporal atrophy, especially the fronto-insular and right frontal structures, and correlates with symptom severity.

If the brain MRI is unremarkable, it is appropriate to consider obtaining a brain scan via fluorodeoxyglucose positron emission tomography (FDG-PET) or perfusion single-photon emission computed tomography (SPECT) if FDG-PET is not available. FDG-PET's advantage over structural imaging is its increased sensitivity, resulting in an early-stage diagnosis. Frontal or temporal lobe atrophy and abnormality patterns raise the diagnostic confidence from possible to probable bvFTD and increase diagnostic specificity from 82% to 95%. Unfortunately, the clinical utility of neuroimaging in bvFTD is limited as the findings do not help alter the disease course, management, or prognosis. CSF analysis can be helpful to rule out AD and rare neurologic conditions. Electroencephalography (EEG) findings in bvFTD are nonspecific and of limited diagnostic value. Finally, a family history of early-onset dementia in first-degree relatives warrants genetic testing for chromosome 9 open reading frame 72 (C9ORF72), granulin precursor (GRN), and microtubule-associated protein tau (MAPT) and a referral for genetic counseling if any of these are positive.

TREATMENT

There are currently no effective disease-modifying treatments to change the course of bvFTD. Nonpharmacologic and pharmacologic interventions are used primarily for symptomatic relief, particularly the behavioral symptoms in bvFTD. Nonpharmacologic interventions are the preferred first-line options and represent the mainstay of management; they should focus on the patient's safety and well-being. Behavioral interventions include caregiver education, environmental modification, social connections, healthy lifestyle changes, mental and physical activity, and occupational, physical, and speech therapy. They prevent disruptive behaviors, provide symptom remission, minimize caregiver distress, and may substitute for psychopharmacology, which may worsen medical comorbidities in the elderly.

Family and caregiver education should involve discussions about potential consequences of impaired patient judgment and supervision of financial matters, including early retirement, limiting credit card access, and management of bank accounts/assets. Providers should recognize caregiver stress as a significant problem that should be addressed by referral to respite care and caregiver support groups. Patients with dementia and their caregivers are vulnerable to abuse. Clinicians must have a low threshold for suspecting and exploring forms of elder abuse, and if there is a concern for the well-being of the patient or caregiver, Adult Protective Services (APS) must be notified. Referral to a driver safety course must be provided, depending on the patient's cognitive and motor findings, and the patient may need to stop driving. Mandatory reporting to local health departments may be required. Caregivers must monitor and prevent hyperorality-associated placement of dangerous inedible objects in the mouth. Physical therapy may help patients with impending motor impairments and parkinsonism mobility problems and minimize fall risk. Regular exercise routines improve mood, cognition, and overall health.

Behavioral modification techniques can help manage problematic behaviors. A behavioral monitoring log can identify triggers. Caregiver support and education on strategies such as redirection, offering simple choices, and distraction can help manage behavioral symptoms. Environmental approaches such as stimulus control, noise reduction, optimizing structured daily activities, and social interaction can reduce anxiety, irritability, and aggression precipitated by external stimuli. A structured environment that minimizes overstimulation can provide stability and predictability for the patient. Providing environmental cues (e.g., laying out clothing, self-care tools) for wanted behaviors and removing cues (car keys) for problem behaviors can be useful.

The pharmacologic management of behavioral symptoms in bvFTD is focused on boosting serotoninergic activity, given the decreased serotonin levels and 5-HT1A/5-HT2A receptors in frontotemporal regions and neuronal loss in the raphe nuclei. All of the selective serotonin reuptake inhibitors (SSRIs) are potentially effective in improving functioning and behavioral symptoms in bvFTD, including disinhibition, impulsivity, irritability, agitation, apathy, stereotypies, compulsive/repetitive behaviors, and hyperorality. Low-dose trazodone can be effective in managing irritability, agitation, aggression, depressive symptoms, and eating disorders.

The neuropathology of bvFTD also causes dopaminergic system disruption with decreased dopamine metabolites and presynaptic dopamine transporters in the putamen and caudate. Dopaminergic medications such as methylphenidate, dextroamphetamine, and bromocriptine are effective in improving risk-taking behaviors, apathy, disinhibition, and speech production. Tetrabenazine can improve severe tics and stereotypies associated with bvFTD. Low-dose atypical antipsychotics such as risperidone, quetiapine, olanzapine, and aripiprazole may help treat both behavioral symptoms and psychosis, either as a substitute for or as an adjunct to SSRIs. Older patients are particularly vulnerable to extrapyramidal side effects, so an agent with relatively low affinity for D2 receptor antagonism such as quetiapine may cause fewer side effects. Frequent monitoring is necessary due to the side effects associated with antipsychotics, which include increased drowsiness, falls, and paradoxical disinhibition.

There is no evidence that a cholinergic deficit is central to the cognitive decline in FTD, and thus no clear benefit from acetylcholinesterase inhibitors (AChEIs) is expected, despite their use in up to 40% of patients with FTD. Donepezil does not seem to help and in fact may make symptoms worse. Similarly, the N-methyl-D-aspartate (NMDA)/glutamate receptor antagonist memantine is well tolerated but has no clear benefits in alleviating bvFTD symptoms or delaying disease progression. Benzodiazepines are often used but can also cause worsening of neurobehavioral symptoms. Neither lithium nor anticonvulsants such as valproate, carbamazepine, topiramate, and lamotrigine have any proven efficacy in managing behavioral symptoms, and the risks of toxicity tend to outweigh the benefits.

- FTD is the third most common form of dementia across all age groups, and the leading cause of early-onset dementia.
- bvFTD, the most common clinical syndrome, is characterized by profound behavioral and neuropsychiatric changes (personality changes, disinhibition, loss of empathy, compulsive/ perseverative behaviors, apathy, dietary changes) mimicking psychiatric disorders.
- A comprehensive clinical assessment incorporating a thorough history, neuropsychological testing, laboratory work-up, neuroimaging, and genetic testing (if indicated) can help accurately diagnose bvFTD in patients presenting with psychiatric symptoms while minimizing misdiagnosis.
- There are no FDA-approved treatments or disease-modifying curative drugs for bvFTD. Nonpharmacologic and pharmacologic interventions provide symptomatic relief by alleviating the severity of behavioral and psychiatric symptoms.

Further Reading

Ducharme S, Price BH, Larvie M, Dougherty DD, Dickerson BC. Clinical approach to the differential diagnosis between behavioral variant frontotemporal dementia and primary psychiatric disorders. *Am J Psychiatry*. 2015;172(9):827–837.

Ferenczi EA, Erkkinen MG, Feany MB, Fogel BS, Daffner KR. New-onset delusions heralding an underlying neurodegenerative condition: A case report and review of the literature. *J Clin Psychiatry*. 2020;81(2):19r13027.

Miller B, Llibre Guerra JJ. Frontotemporal dementia. *Handb Clin Neurol*. 2019;165:33–45.

National Institute on Aging. (2020, June 20). Frontotemporal disorders. https://www. nia.nih.gov/health/topics/frontotemporal-disorders

Woolley JD, Khan BK, Murthy NK, Miller BL, Rankin KP. The diagnostic challenge of psychiatric symptoms in neurodegenerative disease: Rates of and risk factors for prior psychiatric diagnosis in patients with early neurodegenerative disease. *J Clin Psychiatry*. 2011;72(2):126–133.

Younes K, Miller BL. Frontotemporal dementia: Neuropathology, genetics, neuroimaging, and treatments. *Psychiatr Clin North Am*. 2020;43(2):331–344.

12 A telling triad of symptoms

Fanny Huynh Du, Robert T. Hess, and Steve Huege

A 76-year-old male with a history of severe lumbar stenosis and hypertension presented to the clinic for evaluation of 9 months of worsening gait. He initially noticed stiffness in his knees and then began experiencing falls. A few months later, he started to feel as if his feet were stuck to the ground when he was walking. Six months after onset of gait instability, he developed urinary urgency, then incontinence, and struggled to handle his finances. He had to quit working due to symptoms. He scored 20 out of 30 on the Montreal Cognitive Assessment (MoCA), losing points on sections for executive function, attention, language fluency, delayed recall, and orientation. On examination, he had mild proximal leg weakness bilaterally, symmetric hyperreflexia, slowed finger taps, and a wide-based gait with frequent freezing and feet sticking close to the ground. Magnetic resonance imaging (MRI) of the brain revealed ventricular enlargement out of proportion to mild generalized cerebral atrophy.

What do you do now?

This is a patient who is experiencing several months of progressive gait impairment, urinary incontinence, and cognitive deficits that are now impacting his ability to work and perform his instrumental activities of daily living. It would not be unusual for someone of his age to have developed any one or a combination of these symptoms due to a variety of comorbidities and common etiologies. What *is* particularly concerning is his marked decline compared to his baseline functional status. Given the progression of symptoms, a neurodegenerative neurocognitive disorder should be considered. While ventriculomegaly is a common finding in elderly patients due to increasing brain atrophy with age leading to hydrocephalus *ex vacuo*, the patient's enlarged ventricles are disproportionate to his mild atrophy; this presentation is more suggestive of normal pressure hydrocephalus (NPH). NPH is a relatively rare diagnosis among older adults, with median age of onset of 70 years. Prevalence is 0.2% in those aged 70 to 79 and 5.9% in those older than 80 years. NPH accounts for less than 5% of all cases of dementia. It is critical to make an early diagnosis since it is potentially reversible.

DEFINING NPH

NPH is a condition in which there is ventriculomegaly and normal opening pressure on lumbar puncture. It is a form of communicating hydrocephalus. The mechanism of NPH is not fully understood; theories include reduced cerebrospinal fluid (CSF) absorption and reduced ventricular compliance, likely leading to an initial period of increased intracranial pressure (ICP). Over time, the CSF is forced into the periventricular space, causing interstitial edema; the ventricles enlarge; and the ICP eventually normalizes. As a result, neuronal injury may occur due to mechanical stretching of the tracts involved in motor control of the legs and voluntary control of the bladder. Additionally, decreased periventricular blood flow may contribute to neurocognitive impairment.

NPH can produce the classic triad of symptoms often known as "wet, wacky, and wobbly," referring to urinary incontinence, dementia, and gait disturbance. Typically, gait impairment is the first symptom of NPH and also the first symptom to improve with intervention. The characteristic gait of NPH includes shuffling, magnetic gait with feet appearing stuck to the ground, en bloc turning requiring many steps to turn, freezing of gait, and postural instability. The cognitive impairment of NPH involves executive function deficits and apathy. Cortical signs such as prominent language deficits, limb apraxia (in which patients lose the ability to operate devices or tools like phones or remote controls), and impaired short-term memory are uncommon in NPH, and their presence would suggest an alternative diagnosis such as Alzheimer's disease. Rapid eye movement sleep behavior disorder, in which patients act out dreams (can be seen in parkinsonian syndromes), and prominent visual hallucinations (common in dementia with Lewy bodies) do not usually occur in NPH. The urinary symptoms in NPH often begin with urinary urgency, frequency, or nocturia and then progress to incontinence; thus, it is critical not to misdiagnose or attribute these symptoms to a primary urologic condition. Although many patients do not present with the complete classic triad of NPH, gait disturbance is required to diagnose it.

DIAGNOSTIC WORK-UP

A non-contrast computed tomography (CT) scan of the head can effectively assess for ventriculomegaly, and absence of this finding rules out NPH. The imaging of choice, however, is an MRI brain without contrast, which is more sensitive in detecting other signs of NPH. A useful tool for analyzing either form of neuroimaging is the Evans Index, which is the ratio of the widest diameter of the frontal horns compared to the widest diameter of the brain on the same axial slice. An Evans Index of 0.30 or greater, which was the case in this patient (Figure 12.1), is seen in ventriculomegaly and is a criterion for diagnosing NPH. However, ventriculomegaly is not specific for NPH since brain atrophy and other causes of hydrocephalus can similarly have high Evans indices. Hydrocephalus *ex vacuo*, in which the ventricles are enlarged due to brain atrophy, is far more common than NPH in elderly patients. Disproportionately enlarged subarachnoid space hydrocephalus (DESH) is more specific to NPH and is associated with a positive response to shunting. DESH refers to crowding of the sulci superiorly and enlargement of CSF spaces in the sulci inferiorly. These features were seen in this patient's MRI (Figure 12.2).

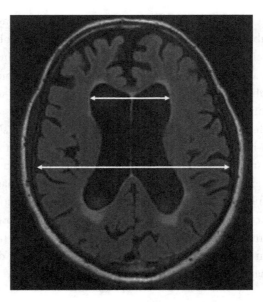

FIGURE 12.1 The patient's Evans Index, calculated as the ratio of the widest diameter of the frontal horns compared to the widest diameter of the brain on the same axial slice of his MRI (*arrows*), is well over 0.30. This indicates ventriculomegaly.

Based on the patient's clinical presentation and MRI, he has a diagnosis of probable NPH. The next test to consider would be large-volume CSF drainage. The patient underwent a lumbar puncture, and his opening pressure was found to be normal at 15 cmH$_2$O, and 40 mL of CSF was removed. He performed several Timed-Up-and-Go (TUG) tests, which involved timing him as soon as he was instructed to get up from a chair and walk 3 meters (10 feet) until he returned to his seat. The TUG test was done before the lumbar puncture as well as 1 hour and 2.5 hours later. Unfortunately, there was no significant change in his gait. In fact, the time he took to complete the test was exactly the same in all trials.

Typically in the evaluation of NPH, at least 30 mL of CSF is removed via lumbar puncture. Another option for CSF removal is placement of an external lumbar drain with steady CSF drainage of 10 to 15 mL per hour for 1 to 3 days or more. A significant improvement, especially in gait and perhaps cognition, after CSF removal confirms the diagnosis of NPH and is strongly

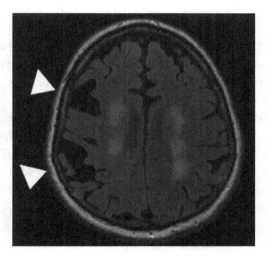

FIGURE 12.2 The patient's MRI brain demonstrates enlarged CSF spaces in these sulci (*arrowheads*), which is referred to as disproportionately enlarged subarachnoid hydrocephalus (DESH) and is a more specific indication of NPH.

associated with a positive response to shunting. While prolonged external lumbar drainage is more sensitive than lumbar puncture, false negatives do occur with both. CSF removal should be accompanied by a pre- and post-intervention gait assessments and perhaps cognitive assessments, depending on the patient's deficits. Aspects of the gait to focus on include total number of steps taken, number of steps needed to turn, and time to complete the test. It is useful to record a video of each gait assessment to provide direct comparisons. A Mini–Mental State Examination (MMSE) or a variety of other cognitive tests can be used.

Besides large-volume CSF drainage, other studies such as MRI CSF flow studies are also sometimes used to predict response to shunting. However, these are still of questionable value, with plenty of false-positive and false-negative results. The patient actually did have an MRI CSF flow study that predicted poor response to shunting. Given the lack of response to CSF removal and based on the MRI CSF flow result, shunting was not pursued at this point. His symptoms continued to worsen. Meanwhile, he had been undergoing a thorough evaluation for other potential contributors to his symptoms.

COMORBID PROBLEMS

It is critical to assess for comorbidities that can lead to or exacerbate symptoms seen in NPH. Regarding gait, performing an assessment for spinal stenosis, neuropathy, osteoarthritis, and orthostatic hypotension would be prudent. With urinary symptoms, assessment for urinary tract infection, prostate enlargement, and functional incontinence should be done. For dementia, other reversible causes such as vitamin B_{12} deficiency, thyroid hormone abnormalities, infectious etiologies such as HIV and syphilis, and other toxic or medication-induced causes should be looked into. Alternative neurodegenerative dementias should be considered as well, although Alzheimer's disease can co-occur in 30% of NPH cases. In addition, cardiovascular risk factors such as hypertension, diabetes, hyperlipidemia, and tobacco smoking can lead to periventricular microvascular ischemia, which can further disturb the flow of CSF and lead to vascular dementia or vascular parkinsonism. These risk factors should be aggressively managed.

The patient underwent MRI of his cervical spine, which showed chronic cervical stenosis, and MRI of his lumbar spine, which showed moderate lumbar stenosis. However, somatosensory evoked potential testing for myelopathy was normal, and a nerve conduction study and electromyography only revealed a length-dependent sensory polyneuropathy without evidence of lumbosacral radiculopathy. A year after onset of symptoms, he now required the use of a walker, his MoCA score had dropped to 18 out of 30, and his urinary incontinence had worsened. He was evaluated by multiple physicians, and his case was discussed at a multidisciplinary team conference. A year and a half after the onset of symptoms, a ventriculoperitoneal (VP) shunt was placed.

TREATMENT

NPH is a potentially reversible cause of dementia. The decision on whether to pursue surgical intervention requires weighing the risks versus benefits. Patients who demonstrate improvement on post-CSF-removal gait assessments are more likely to benefit from VP shunt placement. Patients who do not respond to CSF removal may still respond to VP shunting, but in a lower proportion. Patients who have had symptoms for longer than 2 years or have developed dementia at onset have a lower chance of improvement with VP shunt placement. While ancillary studies can help further stratify surgical candidates, there are no tests that predict a positive response with certainty. In prior decades, complications were more common and included significant risks of mortality, infection, subdural hematoma, seizures, and shunt revision. Complication rates are much lower today, thanks to advancements in surgical techniques and shunt technology, but should still be considered. Those who undergo and respond to surgical intervention appear to have a normal life expectancy compared to those without NPH. Patients undergoing VP shunting are also more likely to regain independence and live independently. The alternative to pursuing surgical intervention is likely continued progression of gait, cognitive, and urinary symptoms, leading to eventual complete loss of independence and early mortality. For these reasons, the benefits and risks of surgery should be carefully considered in all patients with NPH.

Within a month of VP shunt placement, the patient reported improvement in his gait, reduced freezing, improved apathy, and improved urinary incontinence. Six months after shunt placement, he could walk without the use of any assistive devices and was no longer falling. His urinary issues resolved, and his energy levels improved. One year after shunting, he was doing well. Although he was not completely back to his baseline, he continued to notice ongoing gradual improvement.

KEY POINTS TO REMEMBER

- NPH is a relatively rare cause of dementia but one that is important to recognize as it is potentially reversible.
- NPH should be considered in older patients with gait disturbance and either cognitive deficits or urinary incontinence.
- Brain imaging, ideally with MRI brain or CT head, and improvement of gait with CSF removal help to confirm the diagnosis and predict response to shunting.
- Ventriculomegaly is a common finding in the elderly and is not specific for NPH; however, DESH is.
- Comorbidities that can exacerbate dementia, gait disturbance, and urinary incontinence should be thoroughly assessed.

Further Reading

Damasceno BP. Normal pressure hydrocephalus: Diagnostic and predictive
    evaluation. *Dement Neuropsychol.* 2009;3(1):8–15.

Graff-Radford NR, Jones DT. Normal pressure hydrocephalus. *Continuum.*
    2019;25(1):165–186.

Shprecher D, Schwalb J, Kurlan R. Normal pressure hydrocephalus: Diagnosis and
    treatment. *Curr Neurol Neurosci Rep.* 2008;8(5):371–376.

Williams MA, Relkin NR. Diagnosis and management of idiopathic normal-pressure
    hydrocephalus. *Neurol Clin Pract.* 2013;3(5):375–385.

PART III

Anxiety Disorders

13 I'm always afraid

Maria Rueda-Lara and
Elizabeth A. Crocco

A 73-year-old woman with a longstanding history of anxiety presents for a psychiatric evaluation. She was an anxious young girl who suffered from separation anxiety and shyness. Her anxiety worsened after she went to college. Her overall health was generally good, despite a variety of somatic complaints, including headaches and muscle aches. Over the years, her friends and family chided her for "worrying too much." Four years ago, she was diagnosed with stage I breast cancer, and underwent treatment, including a lumpectomy, radiation, and chemotherapy, and is in remission. Her anxiety worsened significantly after her cancer diagnosis. She remains fearful that the cancer might come back somewhere in her body. On one occasion she felt pain on her right earlobe and thought, "My God, cancer came back in my right earlobe!" despite knowing how ridiculous that was. Her fears that her cancer may not allow her to remain independent has affected her ability to enjoy life.

What do you do now?

Anxiety, characterized by excessive worry or fear, manifests itself as a disturbance in mood, thinking, behavior, and physiologic activity for old and young alike. Older adults typically have concerns about their health, loss of independence, family conflicts, and financial issues. Overall, the geriatric population does not suffer from an increased amount of anxiety as compared to the general population. However, patients who have significant comorbidity with psychiatric and medical conditions tend to suffer more from anxiety that is distressing and leads to dysfunction.

PREVALENCE

The prevalence of anxiety in the elderly varies widely. The National Comorbidity Survey Replication (NCS-R) found much lower rates of all anxiety disorders in individuals aged 65 years and older compared with their peak prevalence in individuals aged 18 to 44 years. In contrast, the Longitudinal Aging Study Amsterdam, one of the largest epidemiologic studies to focus on psychiatric disorders in elderly persons, demonstrated that more than 10% of elderly adults had any anxiety disorder, including generalized anxiety disorder (GAD), any phobic disorder, panic disorder, and/or obsessive–compulsive disorder (OCD), which is closer to estimates in younger adults. The discrepancy may be better understood due to the vast variability of prevalence studies and diagnostic criteria. In general, the elderly may suffer from anxiety syndromes that do not meet full criteria for clinical anxiety disorder and therefore may be missed.

CAUSES AND COMORBIDITIES

Anxiety disorders are prevalent in the medically ill and are associated with low levels of health-related quality of life and increased physical disability. In this case, for example, not only does the patient suffer from a chronic life-long anxiety disorder, but her symptoms have been amplified by her medical comorbidities as well as the aging process. It is important to assess the impact of anxiety in all areas of daily functioning when faced with this type of patient. Some are reactions to the stress of a medical illness, whereas others are a consequence of its biologic effects. In the latter case, they are referred to as anxiety disorders due to a medical condition and may be one of the presenting manifestations of a medical disorder. Given this complex interplay between anxiety and illness, it is common in primary care, and in the medical population, anxiety symptoms are significantly higher.

Within the context of cancer, patients may have anxiety related to loss of control, fear of the future, and fear of death. This patient's anxiety worsened after her cancer diagnosis. Some degree of anxiety is experienced by most cancer patients during their course of illness. It presents during crisis points such as initial diagnosis, initiation of treatment, unsuccessful treatment, and cancer recurrence. However, anxiety disorders in older people with cancer have been overlooked as a cause of morbidity. Among older adults with cancer, comorbid medical conditions, frailty, social isolation, poor social support, and fear of worsening physical and cognitive functioning may increase vulnerability to anxiety syndromes. The prevalence of anxiety increases with advanced stage of disease, reduced physical function, and worsening frailty.

In older cancer patients, anxiety is commonly associated with depression. As new medical diseases emerge and treatment is prolonged, patients' anxiety may begin to interfere with their ability to make treatment decisions and adhere to lengthy treatments. An even more serious consequence of anxiety is suicide. The risk of self-harm must be vigorously evaluated in this case, given her amplified negative perception of her illness and sense of hopelessness.

Patients with untreated anxiety make greater use of medical services and have less favorable medical outcomes. Unfortunately, anxiety remains underdiagnosed and providers minimize its importance and consider it a normal response to having an illness. The impact of anxiety symptoms among the medically ill is outlined in Box 13.1. These symptoms can worsen disability and increase mortality. Recognition and treatment are imperative.

GENERALIZED ANXIETY DISORDER

GAD is one of the most common anxiety disorders in the elderly and can be comorbid with other psychiatric conditions. It is characterized by excessive worry or anticipation of future negative events. The anxiety is difficult to control and causes distress. GAD symptoms can vary and include muscle tension, restlessness (or feeling keyed up or on edge), sleeping difficulties, concentration problems, fatigue, and irritability. In addition, low mood is a frequent feature of GAD. Irritability and mood disturbance in this type of patient has led many to believe that the elderly develop unpleasant personalities. This is a myth that leads to the underdiagnosis of both anxiety and mood disorders. GAD tends to be chronic rather than episodic. Because of its chronicity, GAD is one of the least likely mental disorders in the anxiety-affective spectrum to remit spontaneously over time. Other reports have suggested that in elderly persons, chronic GAD tends to develop into a somatization condition or mixed GAD and a major depressive disorder (MDD).

The anxiety in this patient manifested as somatic complaints. Any physical symptoms were magnified and linked to the worst-case scenario. Her physical symptoms always flared up when she was more anxious.

ANXIETY IN THE SETTING OF NEURODEGENERATIVE DISORDERS

Depression and anxiety are very common in people with both major and minor neurocognitive impairment. Additionally, anxiety and depression have a substantial impact on outcomes, as they decrease the ability to live independently, increase the risk of institutionalization, and result in higher caregiver burden. Anxious patients may have more difficulty concentrating. In geriatric patients, it is always important to assess for underlying cognitive deficits, which may not be explained by anxiety alone.

ANXIETY WITH COMORBID DEPRESSION

Patients who have anxiety commonly have comorbid depression. Furthermore, anxiety may be a risk factor for late-life depression. As in this case, although the presenting symptom is anxiety, it is crucial to also evaluate for clinical depression. It is common for patients with depression to be anxious. If the underlying depression is not adequately diagnosed and managed, the patient's symptoms will persist, potentially placing the patient at high risk of self-harm or functional impairment. When depression precedes or is concurrent with the anxiety disorder, anxiety symptoms often persist after remission of depression and increase the risk for depressive relapse. Patients have reduced response rate or delayed response to treatment when anxiety and depression are comorbid. This is an additional reason why the proper diagnosis should be made.

ANXIETY DUE TO ANOTHER MEDICAL CONDITION

Many medical disorders have been reported to cause anxiety. As in this case, elderly patients often have multiple medical comorbidities that may be direct cause of the anxiety symptoms. It is important to consider medical causes of anxiety, particularly when the history is atypical for a primary anxiety disorder (i.e., lack of psychosocial stressors) and when the onset of anxiety is at a later age concomitant with a medical disorder. It is also important to rule out medical causes when the anxiety is accompanied by a disproportionate number of physical symptoms.

Because medical disorders are well known to cause anxiety in the elderly, a full medical evaluation is necessary, even in this patient who has had a life-long anxiety syndrome. The medical evaluation of the anxious patient should begin with a thorough history and physical examination, including neurologic examination. Further components of the evaluation—including laboratory tests, imaging, and other diagnostic studies—should be determined by the patient's specific medical symptoms. For example, a patient with seizure-like episodes will likely require a neurologic consultation and an electroencephalogram. In the absence of other findings suggestive of rare medical etiologies of anxiety, it is not advisable to routinely screen for them (e.g., pheochromocytoma or carcinoid tumors). Table 13.1 depicts common medical conditions associated with anxiety.

TABLE 13.1 **Medical conditions associated with anxiety**

Cardiovascular conditions	Neurologic conditions
Angina pectoris	Akathisia
Arrhythmia	Encephalopathy
Congestive heart failure	Central nervous system mass lesion
Hypovolemia	Post-concussion syndrome
Myocardial infarction	Seizure disorder
Valvular disease	Multiple sclerosis
	Vertigo
Endocrine conditions	Parkinson's disease
Carcinoid	Alzheimer's disease
Hyperadrenalism	
Hypercalcemia	**Gastrointestinal conditions**
Hypothyroidism	Peptic ulcer
Hypocalcemia	
Hyperthyroidism	**Respiratory conditions**
Pheochromocytoma	Asthma
	Chronic obstructive pulmonary disease
Metabolic conditions	Pneumothorax
Hyperkalemia	Pulmonary embolism
Hyperthermia	
Hypoglycemia	**Immunologic conditions**
Hyponatremia	Anaphylaxis
Hypoxia	Systemic lupus erythematosus
Porphyria	

MEDICAL TREATMENTS AND ANXIETY

Treatments such as medication, surgery, radiation, and chemotherapy can cause anxiety in select medical patients. *In this case, the patient received numerous treatment regimens, including surgery, radiation, and chemotherapy. Additionally, she is taking tamoxifen to prevent cancer recurrence. As an example, tamoxifen can cause depression in some patients. Although this patient presented with anxiety, her symptoms may be part of a larger clinical depression.* Table 13.2 displays medications that are commonly associated with anxiety. It is important when evaluating a patient to examine what medications and treatments the patient had recently received in relation to the onset of anxiety symptoms.

TABLE 13.2 **Medications associated with anxiety**

Anesthetics/analgesics	Insulin
Anticonvulsants	Muscle relaxants
Antidepressants	Nonsteroidal anti-inflammatories
Antiemetics	Procaine
Antihistamines	Procarbazine
Antihypertensives	Sedatives
Antimicrobials	Steroids
Antipsychotics	Sympathomimetics
Bronchodilators	Theophylline
Caffeine preparations	Thyroid preparations
Calcium-blocking agents	
Cholinergic-blocking agents	
Digitalis	
Dopaminergic agents (levodopa)	
Ethosuximide	
Hormonal replacement and suppressors	
Hydralazine	
Immunotherapies	

TREATMENT OF SYMPTOMATIC ANXIETY

The primary goals for management of anxiety in geriatric patients include reducing the patient's anxiety and distress and improving overall functioning. It is important to recognize the triggers, presentation, and setting of the anxious symptoms. Other factors include problematic patient behavior such as treatment adherence, as well as the family and staff's negative response to the patient's distress. Anxiety disorders have a waxing and waning course in elderly adults, as in young adults, but these disorders are unlikely to remit completely in older patients. Additionally, anxiety disorders produce quality-of-life impairments and disability on par with that of late-life depression and may be risk factors for the development of depression with anxious distress, a severe and treatment-resistant illness. Treatment is necessary for optimal management of the medically sick patient. The available evidence shows that psychotherapy and pharmacotherapy are most effective combined. Medications alone do not have the same efficacy as a stand-alone treatment.

Psychotherapy

Psychotherapeutic treatment options include psychoeducation and insight-oriented and cognitive-behavioral therapy (CBT). Patients should always be educated about how to recognize their own symptoms of anxiety, factors that trigger or exacerbate them, and the role and efficacy of therapy. CBT is most commonly used in older patients and is primarily aimed at gently but persistently helping patients to recognize automatic yet unrealistic or distorted thoughts that lead to excessive worrying, and then to replace them with more credible and accurate perspectives. Several behavioral approaches that are part of CBT to help in reducing symptoms of anxiety include progressive muscle relaxation (PMR), breathing exercises, meditation, systematic desensitization, exposure and response prevention (a core feature of treating OCD), distraction, guided imagery, and mindfulness. Most older adults with GAD can learn new skills in CBT and use them effectively over time.

Pharmacotherapy

Older adults with GAD often present to primary care or specialty medical care with associated symptoms that may be somatic or neurovegetative. These symptoms often become the targets of treatment, such as using benzodiazepines for sleep, muscle relaxants or even physical therapy referral for muscle tension, and acetylcholinesterase inhibitors for cognitive complaints. These treatments may improve some symptoms in the short term, but they may not treat the underlying anxiety syndrome. Benzodiazepines in particular are highly efficacious in reducing anxiety symptoms, but they carry the risks in older individuals of increasing falls and cognitive impairment. Benzodiazepines can be important medications to reduce acute anxiety but should be selected and dosed carefully and tapered as soon as possible. Preferred benzodiazepines are alprazolam and lorazepam since they have relatively short half-lives and a minimal number of active metabolites.

Antidepressants are considered first-line treatment for anxiety disorders in both young and older adults and include the selective serotonin reuptake inhibitors (SSRIs; fluoxetine, sertraline, paroxetine, citalopram, and escitalopram) and norepinephrine reuptake inhibitors (SNRIs; duloxetine and venlafaxine). SSRIs and SNRIs are all efficacious, can be prescribed in the long term without the risks posed by benzodiazepines, and are better tolerated than the classic medications used for anxiety disorders such as the tricyclic and tetracyclic antidepressants. Clinicians should always initiate medications at no more than half the usual starting dose—sometimes one-fourth or one-eighth, depending on how frail the patient is. In older adults, close consideration of drug–drug interactions is also necessary to prevent unwanted side effects. Titration is necessary but must be done gradually, and side effects must be monitored closely.

KEY POINTS TO REMEMBER

- Both symptomatic anxiety and anxiety disorders are common in older individuals and are often associated with medical conditions as causes and comorbidities. Anxiety is also commonly comorbid with depression and with neurocognitive disorders.
- A thorough history for medical comorbidities and iatrogenic causes is a cornerstone of management.
- Psychotherapeutic approaches, including psychoeducation, insight-oriented therapy, and CBT, should be considered first-line treatment options.
- Antidepressants are considered the first line of medication management. Benzodiazepines, while efficacious in managing acute anxiety, should be used highly cautiously.

Further Reading

Beekman ATF, Bremmer MA, Deeg DJH, Van Balkom AJLM, Smit IH, De Beurs E, Van Dyck R, Van Tilburg W. Anxiety disorders in later life: A report from the Longitudinal Aging Study Amsterdam. *Int J Geriatr Psychiatry*. 1998;13(10):717–726.

Ferreti L, McCurry SM, Logsdon R, Gibbons L, Teri L. Anxiety and Alzheimer's disease. *J Geriatr Psychiatry Neurol*. 2001;14:52–58.

Gum AM, Petkus A, McDougal SJ, Present M, King-Kallimanis B, Schonfeld L. Behavioral health needs and problem recognition by older adults receiving home-based aging services. *Int J Geriatr Psychiatry*. 2009;24(4):400–408.

14 I felt as though I was about to die

Rachel Zack Ishikawa and Feyza Marouf

A 75-year-old man with moderate, stable chronic obstructive pulmonary disease (COPD) and a longstanding history of worrying that is hard to control describes "spells" marked by shortness of breath, chest pain, rapid heart rate, sweating, and fear of death. Over time, fear of these symptoms led to increased isolation. The patient stopped seeing friends over the past month and is not driving more than a few miles from his home because he fears having a spell while driving. The sensation of breathlessness is particularly difficult for him to tolerate. He worries that he might suffer a stroke or heart attack when the episodes occur. His primary care doctor prescribed an albuterol inhaler for management of COPD, and he recently started lorazepam twice daily for these episodes. He views the lorazepam as critical for symptom management and is mistrustful of any changes to his regimen.

What do you do now?

Anxiety disorders are often underdiagnosed among older adults, with more than two-thirds of adults with late-life anxiety receiving no treatment. Careful evaluation is critical for diagnostic clarity and identification of appropriate treatment. In this case, the pattern of frequent, multi-symptom episodes, fear of future attacks, and behavioral avoidance suggests a diagnosis of panic disorder (PD). Panic attacks may be distinguished from other anxiety symptoms by their primarily somatic nature. In addition to the reported panic symptoms, this patient reports worry that is hard to control, which is a hallmark symptom of generalized anxiety disorder. PD is the second most prevalent anxiety disorder among older adults, after agoraphobia, with an estimated 12-month prevalence ranging from 0.7% to 3.6% among adults over the age of 65. The prevalence is lower than that found among younger adults (4.7%). Most older adults developed panic disorder in younger adulthood, with less than 1% developing panic disorder after age 62.

WHAT ARE PANIC ATTACKS?

A panic attack is an abrupt surge of intense fear or intense discomfort that reaches a peak within minutes. Symptoms typically escalate rapidly, and are characterized by sympathetic nervous system activation, accompanied by intense fear of loss of control, heart attack, or death (Box 14.1). It may occur suddenly, or appear in response to acute stressors. PD is characterized by a history of recurrent and unexpected panic attacks, and involves persistent concern or worry about additional panic attacks or their consequences, such as losing control, having a heart attack, or having a cardiac event far from home or emergency medical care. It often leads to a significant and maladaptive change in behavior related to the attacks, such as avoidance of exercise or unfamiliar situations, or agoraphobic avoidance.

The symptoms of PD must be distinguished from the physiologic effects of a substance or another medical condition or mental disorder. For example, symptoms of a panic attack are sometimes indistinguishable from an actual cardiac event, especially in individuals with preexisting cardiac conditions. Symptoms common to both panic and COPD include hyperventilation, chest tension, dizziness, lightheadedness, air hunger, and fear of death. In the opening case, the man has COPD and can't distinguish between dyspnea and panic attacks. In addition, he may be at increased risk for more severe cardiopulmonary complications as a result of panic, as well as being more likely to panic in response to chest pain or restriction in his breathing.

In PD, patients become hypervigilant to interoceptive sensations, or the internal physiologic state of the body. Interoceptive sensitivity, together with cognitive interpretations of physiologic sensations as potentially threatening, elicit the "fear of fear" cycle, wherein patients interpret as dangerous not only the symptoms but also the fear about the symptoms themselves. This reaction is heightened in individuals with COPD, because worsening dyspnea may signal a potentially fatal attack. This compounding of fear indicates that the individual remains in danger, increasing activation of the sympathetic branch of the autonomic nervous systems, which further heightens the fight-or-flight response. Thus, the panic escalates. Often, the individual tries to "escape" the panic attack by leaving the activating environment or situation, or avoiding it altogether, as with this patient. While this ameliorates panic in the short term, in the long term it reinforces the misattribution that the situation itself is dangerous, and increases the likelihood of future panic attacks. For clinicians it may be helpful to educate patients about this physiologic cascade that triggers panic attacks.

PD symptoms differ between older and younger adults. Compared with younger adults, older adults with PD report fewer and less severe panic symptoms (possibly due to a less active autonomic nervous system); less anxiety, arousal, and depression; and higher levels of functioning. Among older adults who are retired or socially isolative, the impairment or avoidance criteria may be less apparent. Nonetheless, PD is deleterious to older adults' health, contributing to isolation, sedentary behaviors, and high medical service utilization.

APPROACHES TO TREATMENT

Despite the intensity and debilitating nature of its symptoms, PD is eminently treatable, ideally with a combination of psychotherapy and pharmacotherapy. As will be described, individuals find panic attacks so distressing that short-term medications are often needed while waiting for other approaches to work to prevent attacks in the first place.

Cognitive–Behavioral Therapy

The most empirically supported psychotherapeutic treatment for PD is cognitive–behavioral therapy (CBT) that combines repeated and controlled exposure to autonomic physical sensations along with cognitive and somatic coping strategies. These structured exposures allow the individual to habituate to physiologic cues and deactivate the heightened fight-or-flight response. A relevant meta-analysis showed that among the various strategies used in CBT for PD, cognitive restructuring and interoceptive exposure have the greatest impact on treatment effectiveness, while commonly included components such as breathing retraining, muscle relaxation, in vivo exposures, and virtual reality exposures were associated with lower effectiveness. A sample five- to seven-session weekly CBT treatment plan for the 75 year-old man in the case is outlined in Table 14.1.

TABLE 14.1 **A sample CBT treatment plan**

Session(s)	Therapeutic activities/exercises
1	You present the rationale for CBT, explaining the function and procedures of cognitive restructuring and exposure-based treatment. You use a motivational interviewing approach to address the patient's hesitation about discontinuing medications and his fears that exposure therapy will elicit a panic attack or pulmonary complications.
2	You introduce the patient to the CBT model of emotion, which posits that all emotions have physical, emotional, cognitive, and behavioral elements. Thoughts include a sense of doom when he first notices the onset of the attack and fears of needing oxygen, having a heart attack, dying, or being embarrassed if others see his panic attack. You explain to the patient the interconnection between physical sensations and automatic thoughts by illustrating the cycle of panic. Initially, the patient senses subtle physical changes, perhaps a tightness in his chest after climbing a flight of stairs. Because of his interoceptive sensitivity, he is highly attuned to these sensations, and immediately interprets them as worrisome and potentially dangerous, thus inviting a cascade of fearful, automatic thoughts. This cognitive engagement then triggers more symptoms, leading to a full panic attack. In response, he searches for an escape, perhaps believing that certain situations (e.g., being far from home, exercising) are themselves dangerous. You explain to him that because of this fear conditioning, he becomes more likely to have a panic attack in similar situations in the future.
3	You introduce the skill of cognitive restructuring, which involves identifying the unhelpful automatic thoughts and challenging their accuracy using specific questions: What is the likely outcome if I have a panic attack? How is someone likely to react if they see me have a panic attack? What is the worst that will happen? If I start to have an attack in the car, what will I do? The answers to these questions help to de-catastrophize the feared outcomes, and remind the patient of the internal and external resources available to him in the event of an attack. Next, you address the patient's automatic thoughts around the difficulty distinguishing COPD symptoms from panic symptoms. You work with the patient to create a "cheat sheet" comparing COPD and PD-related symptoms, such as dyspnea and hyperventilation.

Continued

TABLE 14.1 **Continued**

Session(s)	Therapeutic activities/exercises
4–7	The final sessions are dedicated to interoceptive exposures. You identify exposures that mimic the sensations of panic attacks for this patient, such as restrictive breathing through a narrow straw, jogging in place, or taking deep breaths while pressing on his chest. While engaging in daily exposure practice, the patient uses cognitive restructuring skills to de-catastrophize the physiologic sensations, observing them without anticipating an incipient panic attack. He also reviews his "cheat sheet" to remind himself that he can in fact distinguish between panic and pulmonary symptoms. Lastly, he engages in behavioral exposures to target avoided activities, such as traveling increasing distances from home and reconnecting with friends. He prefers to keep a supply of a benzodiazepine available on an as-needed basis "just in case," but after 6 months he reports that he has only used the medication once. He learns that the most effective way to cope with a panic attack is not to panic about the attack itself, or to rely on medication to quiet the symptoms, but rather to do nothing. He learns to observe the sensations, de-catastrophize his thinking, and wait for the sensations to pass, which they do.

Psychopharmacology

First-line medications for late-life anxiety include the selective serotonin reuptake inhibitors (SSRIs) and the serotonin–norepinephrine reuptake inhibitors (SNRIs). The evidence base for these medications in older adults is limited to small studies of generalized anxiety, PD, and mixed populations. Positive effects compared with placebo have been shown for paroxetine, sertraline, citalopram, escitalopram, venlafaxine, and duloxetine. Two small studies focused on late-life PD found evidence for the superiority of escitalopram over citalopram in time to response. Older individuals generally tolerate SSRIs and SNRIs well, but compared to younger age groups are more susceptible to gait impairment, falls, gastrointestinal bleeds, bone loss, and hyponatremia. The need for treatment based on the severity and duration of symptoms should be weighed carefully against the risks of potential side effects, including anticholinergic (urinary retention, cognitive impairment), antiadrenergic (orthostatic hypotension), and antihistaminergic (sedation) effects.

When there is limited response to an SSRI or SNRI, other serotonergic medications can be considered, including mirtazapine, trazodone, nortriptyline, and buspirone. Sedating antidepressants like mirtazapine and trazodone can be useful for concurrent insomnia. Tricyclics can be particularly effective for people with neuralgias and migraines, but they are not often used in late life due to their strong anticholinergic and orthostatic effects, as well as the risk for slowed cardiac conduction. Studies of buspirone show it is well tolerated in the elderly, and less likely to interact with other medications, but it's best used for generalized anxiety or to augment another antidepressant. Antipsychotic medications like quetiapine, risperidone, olanzapine, and aripiprazole are sometimes used for severe anxiety and even panic, either alone or in combination with an antidepressant, but they are not indicated specifically for PD and can be complicated by their side-effect burden. There are other pharmacologic strategies that have limited efficacy for PD and pose an increased risk of side effects in older individuals, including anticonvulsants (gabapentin, lamotrigine, and topiramate), propranolol, prazosin, and clonidine.

Benzodiazepine use is still exceedingly common among older adults, including those with PD. In fact, 50% of older adults with PD are prescribed these medications. For a patient in high distress, benzodiazepines will take effect immediately and can be used as a "bridge" medication for weeks until an antidepressant begins to alleviate anxiety. They can also be used on an as-needed basis to cover breakthrough symptoms. However, studies show that they are frequently prescribed as monotherapy in the absence of an antidepressant. Unfortunately, older adults are much more sensitive to this class of medications due to age-related alterations in their distribution and elimination as well as increased sensitivity of central nervous system (CNS) receptors to their effects. In older patients benzodiazepines pose an increased risk of causing excess sedation, confusion, unsteadiness, motor instability, and falls. They can also cause paradoxical agitation and disinhibition.

When benzodiazepine therapy becomes necessary for an older patient due to severe or refractory panic symptoms, the preferred choices are short-acting agents such as lorazepam that either lack metabolites or have active compounds that rapidly disappear, and are thus are less likely to accumulate in the body and cause side effects. These agents and their dosing are listed

TABLE 14.2 **Short-acting benzodiazepines used for panic attacks**

Benzodiazepine	Dosage	Half-life	Rate of Onset
Lorazepam	0.5–2 mg	10–20 hours	Intermediate
Oxazepam	15–30 mg	4–15 hours	Slow
Alprazolam	0.25–1 mg	6–12 hours	Intermediate

in Table 14.2. Using the lowest possible doses and minimizing the duration of use helps to reduce the potential for abuse and dependence.

Benzodiazepines are CNS depressants, so care must be taken when combining them with other depressants given the risks of hypotension, sedation, respiratory depression, and death. Commonly, anxious older adults have comorbid substance use disorders, including misuse of alcohol and opiates. Combining benzodiazepines with alcohol can result in harmful disinhibition and retrograde amnesia. Mixing benzodiazepines with opiates can cause lethal respiratory depression. Ketamine, barbiturates, melatonin, tramadol, and pramipexole can also cause major interactions with benzodiazepines, resulting in respiratory depression. Medications such as methylphenidate, pseudoephedrine, phenylephrine, and caffeine antagonize the effects of benzodiazepines, leading to increased benzodiazepine use to counter the stimulants.

The process of tapering a benzodiazepine in older adults can be complex. Fear of withdrawal symptoms or recurrence of anxiety can lead to hesitation about reducing these medications. Successful efforts often begin with strong physician rapport and encouragement, with initial visits focused on patient education about the expected benefits (improved alertness, cognition, gait stability) as well as the risks of long-term use. Clinicians can increase patient motivation by suggesting a trial dose reduction, helping to ease anticipatory anxiety about further reductions. Tapers are best done slowly, often over months rather than weeks, to improve tolerability. Initial reductions in benzodiazepine dose by 25% every few weeks may be adjusted to smaller reductions toward the last quarter of a taper, when withdrawal symptoms tend to be most severe. Tapers that go longer than 6 months are often complicated by preoccupations with the tapering process itself.

As part of the initial treatment plan, you discuss a lorazepam taper with your patient. You explain that because benzodiazepines diminish anxiety/panic reactions, they can reduce the efficacy of interoceptive exposures. This impedes the process of new learning and makes it likely that the patient will not receive the full benefit of treatment. The patient cautiously agrees to taper his use of benzodiazepines while starting an SSRI, although he expresses apprehension about this plan. However, his panic attacks are significantly improved after 6 weeks of taking an SSRI combined with CBT.

KEY POINTS TO REMEMBER

- PD is prevalent among older adults, but diagnosis may be complicated by a symptom profile that overlaps with common medical illnesses.
- CBT is an effective treatment for PD among older adults.
- SSRI antidepressants are considered first-line treatments for PD. Although benzodiazepines are the most common psychopharmacologic treatment prescribed for PD, they carry risks for older adults and are best used to treat acute panic while waiting for the effects of an antidepressant to kick in.

Further Reading
Andreescu C, Varon D. New research on anxiety disorders in the elderly and an update on evidence-based treatments. *Curr Psychiat Rep.* 2015;17(7):53.
Benítez CIP, Smith K, Vasile RG, Rende R, Edelen MO, Keller MB. Use of benzodiazepines and selective serotonin reuptake inhibitors in middle-aged and older adults with anxiety disorders: A longitudinal and prospective study. *Am J Geriatric Psychiatry.* 2008;16(1):5–13.
Meuret AE, Kroll J, Ritz T. Panic disorder comorbidity with medical conditions and treatment implications. *Annu Rev Clin Psycho.* 2017;13(1):209–240.
Pompoli A, Furukawa TA, Imai H, Tajika A, Efthimiou O, Salanti G. Psychological therapies for panic disorder with or without agoraphobia in adults: A network meta-analysis. *Cochrane Database Syst Rev.* 2016;4(4):CD011004.
Tannenbaum C. Inappropriate benzodiazepine use in elderly patients and its reduction. *J Psychiatr Neurosci.* 2015;40(3):E27–E28.
Willgoss TG, Yohannes AM. Anxiety disorders in patients with chronic obstructive pulmonary disease: A systematic review. *Respir Care.* 2012;58(5):858–866.

15 I can't get those thoughts out of my head

Kalya Vardi

A 70-year-old woman presents to your office with her adult daughter. The woman appears tearful and anxious. She explains that since her husband's sudden death 6 months ago, she has been "an anxious wreck." The daughter notes that her mother was functioning well before her husband's death but became sad and anxious since. To her daughter, the woman's symptoms seemed like a normal reaction to the situation. The woman is a practicing lifelong Catholic but about 2 months ago, she abruptly stopped attending her church and would not say why. When her daughter brings up the church, the woman becomes distraught, begging her daughter, "Please don't make me talk about that." You ask to speak with the woman privately. Once alone, the woman adamantly denies that anyone at the church has harmed or threatened her, or otherwise made her feel uncomfortable or unsafe. She explains, "It's not them—I'm the problem. I can't discuss these evil thoughts in my head when my family are around."

What do you do now?

Patients with obsessive–compulsive disorder (OCD) often experience tremendous shame about their symptoms and try to hide them from others. This shame may also prevent them from seeking help. Although the estimated prevalence of OCD is 1% to 3%, many providers do not screen for obsessions or compulsions as part of an initial evaluation. Some studies suggest that the prevalence of OCD has been underestimated because patients do not report their symptoms.

OCD is characterized by the presence of both obsessions and compulsions. Obsessions are recurrent, intrusive thoughts, urges, or images that cause significant distress. Compulsions are repetitive behaviors or mental rituals that the person performs to reduce that distress. To meet the criteria for OCD outlined in the fifth edition of the American Psychiatric Association's *Diagnostic and Statistical Manual of Mental Disorders* (DSM-5), the obsessions and compulsions must be time-consuming, cause clinically significant distress, or impair functioning. If clinical features support a diagnosis, clinicians may consider screening the patient for OCD using the Dimensional Obsessive-Compulsive Scale (DOCS), a self-report questionnaire with 20 items. The DOCS has four subscales, each focusing on a common subtype of OCD symptoms: concerns about contamination, concerns about being responsible for harm, concerns about symmetry or wanting things to be "just right," and unacceptable (taboo) thoughts. If, for example, a patient scores highly in the areas of concerns about causing harm and having unacceptable thoughts, it demonstrates how using a screening tool can help identify the patient's OCD symptoms and create an opening for clinicians to educate patients about OCD, normalize the experience as a medical condition, and offer hope that they may benefit from treatment.

The patient explains that she has a longstanding fear of making errors in daily activities, which has manifested in different ways at different times of her life. In recent years, the patient has had frequent intrusive worries that she made a medication error. The patient fears that she will accidentally overdose on her medications and have a serious adverse event or die. She manages her own medications using a pill box and accurately recalls her medication regimen. To ease her anxiety, the patient compulsively checks her pill box to make sure that she took the medication for that day and did not take the pills from any other days. When her husband was alive, she would ask him to observe her taking her pills and then would seek reassurance from him throughout the day. Since her husband died, the frequency and intensity of her obsessions and compulsions have increased. She estimates that she spends more than an hour checking her pill box each morning and often returns to check it again later in the day.

Despite these symptoms, the patient felt she was managing well enough until 2 months ago. She was keeping busy with activities at her church and found a lot of comfort in prayer and in the support of the church community. Then, one night she awoke from a dream in which she was kissing her priest. Since then, the patient has been having frequent intrusive images of herself kissing her priest, as well as intrusive thoughts that she is a sinner and that she will go to Hell. Although she has no desire to kiss her priest, she is worried that she will, so she stopped going to church to avoid seeing him. To reduce her distress, she says the Lord's Prayer aloud, which provides some relief but not much. She is sleeping poorly, her appetite has declined, and she has lost more than 10 pounds. She avoids talking to friends and family because she does not want to reveal what is going on for fear that they will judge her and cut her out of their lives.

DIAGNOSIS

The woman has never been diagnosed with any psychiatric disorder or received any mental health treatment. The typical age of onset for OCD is teens to 20s, although OCD can occur in children younger than 10 years old. Initial onset after age 50 is exceedingly rare and is usually associated with a neurologic illness or injury. Unfortunately, little research has been done on the epidemiology, diagnosis, or treatment of OCD in older adults. In this case, the patient alludes to a long history of OCD symptoms but struggles to provide details, at least in part due to her current distress. Although undiagnosed, it seems likely that she has a prior history of OCD. However, given her age, it is important to assess for neurologic problems that can manifest with obsessions and compulsions, such as Parkinson's disease, frontotemporal dementia, and strokes in the frontal lobes or basal ganglia.

You perform a neurologic exam and find no focal deficits, rigidity, or tremor. You administer a cognitive screening test, the Montreal Cognitive Assessment (MoCA), and the patient scores 30/30, which indicates that a neurocognitive disorder is unlikely. You refer the patient for magnetic resonance imaging (MRI) of her brain. When you obtain the results, you find no significant abnormalities that would explain her symptoms. So, it is most likely that her current symptoms are attributable to OCD. Fortunately, she denies having any suicidal ideation. She also identifies her daughter and her religious beliefs as reasons to live.

Most patients with OCD have at least one other comorbid psychiatric disorder. In this case, a careful history reveals that the patient also meets the criteria for generalized anxiety disorder (GAD). Importantly, OCD is a risk factor for suicide, with some studies estimating that as many as 25% of people with OCD will attempt suicide in their lifetime.

TREATMENT

The twin pillars of OCD treatment are exposure and response prevention (ERP) and serotonergic medication. ERP is a type of cognitive–behavioral therapy in which patients make a hierarchy of feared situations and then gradually confront them without engaging in compulsions. ERP is designed to challenge the patient's negative assumptions about the feared situation, as well as demonstrate to the patient that the anxiety itself is not dangerous. For ERP to be effective, the patient should experience anxiety and discomfort during the exposure. When ERP is done correctly, patients learn that their worst fears are not realized, and that the distress they experience in a feared situation will naturally diminish over time, even when they stay in the situation and do not engage in compulsions. There is robust research documenting the efficacy of ERP in the general adult population. There are case reports that support its use in older adults with OCD.

You strongly encourage your patient to engage in ERP because the response to treatment with ERP alone is greater than the response to medication alone and comparable to the response to the combination of medication and ERP. You also explain that older adults are more likely to have side effects from medications, which could be reduced or avoided by participating ERP.

Although ERP is considered the gold standard in psychotherapy for OCD, many patients also benefit from learning cognitive strategies to correct maladaptive beliefs and mindfulness skills to manage the physical symptoms of anxiety-related hyperarousal. Cognitive therapy (CT) focuses on cognitive restructuring, which involves identifying and questioning problematic thoughts to develop a more rational and helpful perspective.

Mindfulness means staying focused on the present moment, aware of your thoughts and feelings but not judging them. Mindfulness exercises often use an activity as an anchor to focus on, like deep breathing, progressive muscle relaxation, or coloring mandalas (detailed geometric designs with symbolic meaning in Buddhist and Hindu cultures). Meditation is a type of mindfulness practice.

Mindfulness-based cognitive therapy (MBCT) is a manualized psychotherapy that incorporates mindfulness and CT. Patients who are unwilling to try ERP or who have residual symptoms after ERP should be offered CT or MBCT. In practice, these modalities are often combined.

As previously noted, there is some research demonstrating that cognitively intact older adults can benefit from CBT, including ERP. However, even normal aging is associated with changes in cognition, in particular decreased processing speed and difficulty inhibiting distractions, multitasking, or switching tasks. So, providers who work with older adults should be attentive to potential barriers to learning new concepts and skills, and make adaptations as needed. For example, providers may need to present information more slowly or review concepts more frequently. Providers should limit distractions and may need to narrow the focus on each treatment session. Patients may also benefit from taking notes or making recordings of sessions. In some situations, and only if the patient consents, it may be helpful to involve a family member or caregiver in treatment sessions, so that this supportive person can learn the therapeutic concepts and skills and then help the patient practice them at home. Studies suggest that patients with mild neurocognitive disorder and mild dementia can also benefit from CBT when appropriate modifications are made. Patients with moderate to severe cognitive impairment are unlikely to benefit.

There is little research examining pharmacologic treatment for OCD in older adults. In this context, treatment recommendations are based on results from the general adult population with modifications based on the higher risks of using certain medications in older adults (Table 15.1). Selective serotonin reuptake inhibitors (SSRIs) are first-line medications in the pharmacologic treatment of OCD in the general population and for older adults. Among the SSRIs, sertraline and escitalopram are the most senior-friendly because they are the least likely to cause side effects and drug interactions. Fluoxetine and fluvoxamine are reasonable but second-line

TABLE 15.1 **Pharmacotherapy for OCD in older adults**

	Drug name	Dose range (mg/day)
First line	Escitalopram	2.5–20
	Sertraline	25–400
Second line	Fluoxetine	10–80
	Fluvoxamine	25–300
	Mirtazapine	7.5–60
	Venlafaxine	37.5–375
Third line	Clomipramine	25–250
	Augmenting an SSRI with:	
	· Aripiprazole	2–15
	· Olanzapine	2.5–20
	· Risperidone	0.5–2
	· Other: second antidepressant, other antipsychotic, topiramate, lamotrigine, buspirone	

options for older adults. Fluoxetine has a long half-life and an active metabolite, so older adults who have age- or disease-related declines in liver and kidney function would be more susceptible to toxicity. Fluvoxamine is a potent inhibitor of CYP1A2 and CYP2C9, and it also inhibits CYP2C19 and CYP3A4, so there is a substantial risk of drug interactions. Most notably, warfarin is metabolized by CYP1A2 and CYP2C9, and several common antihypertensives—carvedilol, irbesartan, and losartan—are metabolized by CYP2C9. Escitalopram is preferred over citalopram because the U.S. Food and Drug Administration (FDA) warns that citalopram causes dose-dependent QTc prolongation and recommends a maximum citalopram dose of 20 mg/day in patients over 60 years old. Escitalopram (the S-isomer of citalopram) does not carry the same warning or dosing recommendation because studies suggest that the risk of QTc prolongation is substantially higher with citalopram. Paroxetine is relatively contraindicated in older adults because of potential anticholinergic effects.

If an SSRI is ineffective or poorly tolerated, there is some evidence to support treatment with mirtazapine or venlafaxine, both of which are also reasonably safe for older adults, depending on the patient's comorbidities and other medications. Tricyclic antidepressants, like clomipramine, should be used with caution in older adults due to the risks of arrhythmia, orthostasis, and delirium. Adjunctive treatment with an atypical antipsychotic like risperidone, aripiprazole, or olanzapine can be helpful. However, antipsychotics carry substantial risks, especially in older adults, who are more likely to have comorbidities and polypharmacy. Notably, extrapyramidal side effects are more common in older adults than younger adults. The choice between switching to clomipramine or augmenting an SSRI with an atypical antipsychotic should be based on a thorough review of the patient's risk factors, as well as patient preference (after education about the risks). Other treatment options include combining two antidepressants (including an SSRI and clomipramine) or augmenting with an anticonvulsant medication (like topiramate or lamotrigine). Benzodiazepines should be avoided since there is little evidence that they are helpful in treating OCD and they carry substantial risks in older adults, including a high risk of falls and delirium.

Your patient wants to try the combination of ERP and medication. You prescribe a low dose of sertraline to minimize the risk of side effects and give the patient instructions to increase the dose after 1 week if tolerated. You explain that antidepressant medications work gradually and that response times may be longer for OCD compared to other anxiety or mood disorders and for older adults.

It can take up to 12 weeks to see the full effect of starting an antidepressant or increasing the dose, and it often takes higher doses of antidepressant medication to treat OCD compared to depression or other anxiety disorders. In fact, some patients with OCD will benefit from titrating the antidepressant dose above the FDA-approved maximum. That said, older adults as a group tend to respond to lower doses of medication and tend to have more side effects, so the patient may not need or may not be able to tolerate a higher dose. Dose titration is based on the patient's response to the medication rather than a specific dose or blood level.

For prognostic tracking, the most frequently used instrument is the Yale–Brown Obsessive Compulsive Scale (Y-BOCS). The Y-BOCS is a 10-item clinician-administered scale to quantify the severity of obsessions and compulsions over the prior week. It is the most frequently used outcome measure in OCD research. While the DOCS is useful in screening for OCD symptoms, the Y-BOCS is more appropriate for monitoring symptom severity and treatment response

The patient follows through with the referral for ERP and the medication trial. Over the following months, you titrate the medication dose two more times to target residual symptoms. The patient tolerates the medication well. With the combination of ERP and medication, the patient's OCD symptoms decrease substantially. The obsessions decrease but do not resolve. The taboo images still intrude into her awareness at times, but she recognizes that they are separate from her true beliefs and wishes, and that it is exceedingly unlikely that she would behave in that way. Her functioning improves and she gradually resumes attending Mass and participating in church activities. She finds it harder to extinguish the fear of making a medication error, but she succeeds in reducing the amount of time she spends checking her pill box down to 30 minutes each day. You discuss the possibility of increasing the antidepressant dose further to reduce her symptoms. The patient feels that the symptoms are manageable at the current dose and prefers not to take on any additional risk by increasing the dose. You recommend that she continue the current dose for 1 to 2 years before attempting a taper to minimize the risk of recurrence.

KEY POINTS TO REMEMBER

- Many patients will not spontaneously report obsessions or compulsions due to fear and shame.
- Initial onset of OCD after age 50 is exceedingly rare and is usually associated with a neurologic illness or injury.
- ERP is the most effective treatment for OCD.
- Serotonergic medications also play a key role in treating OCD in late life, especially when combined with ERP. They often take longer to work in older adults, and higher doses are needed to treat OCD compared to other anxiety and depressive disorders.

Further Reading

Jazi AN, Asghar-Ali AA. Obsessive-compulsive disorder in older adults: A comprehensive literature review. *J Psychiatric Practice*. 2020;26(3):175–184.

Jones MK, Wootton BM, Vaccaro LD. The efficacy of exposure and response prevention for geriatric obsessive compulsive disorder: A clinical case illustration. *Case Rep Psychiatry*. 2012;12:1–5.

Katzman MA, Bleau P, Blier P, Chokka P, Kjernisted K, Van Ameringen M; the
    Canadian Anxiety Guidelines Initiative Group on behalf of the Anxiety Disorders
    Association of Canada/Association Canadienne des troubles anxieux and McGill
    University. Canadian clinical practice guidelines for the management of anxiety,
    posttraumatic stress and obsessive-compulsive disorders. *BMC Psychiatry*.
    2014;14(S1):1–83.

16 Every reminder throws me off

Azziza O. Bankole

A 77-year-old woman comes into the clinic with her husband. She is quite anxious and remained so through most of the visit. She reported that her symptoms began about a year ago when the water heater in her home was changed. There was an issue with its installation and she suffered from carbon monoxide poisoning. Since then she has reported waking up in the middle of the night with a burning sensation in her chest and mouth. In addition, she reported having significant anxiety symptoms which lessened when she left her house and increased whenever she was coming back home. Her appetite had been poor. She was depressed and reported impaired self-care, poor motivation, anhedonia, and passive thoughts of death. She has persistent obsessive thoughts about the water heater at home, which had since been replaced. Her husband reported that she had irritable mood and outbursts of anger, affecting her relationships.

What do you do now?

Post-traumatic stress disorder (PTSD) is defined by a cluster of symptoms that occur in response to being exposed to an actual or potential life-threatening injury or event, or sexual violence. Although PTSD is most often discussed within the context of war or conflict, most cases have other causes. In the United States, PTSD is reported in 6.5% of older adults, representing a slight decline from younger cohorts. The basic diagnostic features of PTSD include exposure to a traumatic event, intrusive re-experiencing of the event, avoidance of things that trigger memories of the event, negative thoughts and emotions, and increased arousal or hypervigilant states. To meet criteria for PTSD, these symptoms last for at least 6 months and cause significant functional impairment. These symptoms are described in more detail in Table 16.1, along with the patient's symptoms in the case example.

The diagnosis of PTSD can also be specified for the presence of dissociative symptoms (depersonalization or derealization) and with delayed expression in which the patient does not meet full criteria until at least

TABLE 16.1 **PTSD symptoms according to DSM-5 and in the case example**

Symptom	Patient's symptoms
Exposure Actual or threatened death, serious injury, or sexual violence directly, as a witness, through learning about it occurring to a close family or friend, or through repeated or extreme exposure to aversive details of the traumatic event	Direct exposure to a life-threatening situation with carbon monoxide poisoning. In addition, her husband of almost 60 years was also exposed to the same threat.
Re-experiencing Recurrent, involuntary, and intrusive distressing memories, dreams, flashbacks of the trauma, and/or intense psychological distress and/or physiologic reactions to cues or triggers that symbolize or resemble the trauma	Continuing re-experiencing of the trauma and associated emotional distress over the fact that it happened to her in her own home. Her sleep is impaired, and although she did not report having any nightmares, she had been having frequent nighttime awakenings with a burning sensation in her chest and mouth.

TABLE 16.1 **Continued**

Symptom	Patient's symptoms
Avoidance Efforts made to avoid distressing memories, thoughts, or feelings associated with the trauma and/or to avoid people, places, or circumstances that trigger them	Patient was distressed at home, but her distress decreased when she was away from home. Because the traumatic event happened at home, avoidance is largely difficult for her to maintain.
Negative cognitions and mood Inability to recall part of trauma; distorted and negative self-image or self-blame; fear, anger, guilt; diminished interest in activities and relationships; inability to feel positive, happy, or loving	Anhedonia, fearfulness, and thoughts that her life was no longer worth living were present.
Arousal Irritability; angry outbursts; recklessness; hypervigilance; quick to startle; problems with concentration and sleep	Husband reported that she was having difficulty with irritability of mood and outbursts of anger since the incident. Her sleep was impaired, as mentioned earlier.
Duration Greater than 1 month	Symptoms have been present for 12 months, significantly longer than the required 6 months.
Functional impairment Significant impairment in social, occupational, and other areas of function	Symptoms have caused her significant distress and functional impairment, including a 3-week inpatient psychiatric hospitalization.
Exclusions Symptoms are not attributable to a different condition	Other potential causes of the patient's symptoms such as prescribed and over-the-counter medications, illicit substances, and other medical illnesses were excluded based on her history, collateral information, lab work, and neuroimaging.

6 months after the inciting incident, but may have had some symptoms immediately after the trauma.

PTSD increases an individual's risk of developing comorbid psychiatric disorders, including depression, anxiety disorders, substance use disorders, cognitive decline, and major neurocognitive disorders. There is also an increased risk of suicide. In the case, the patient currently meets the criteria specified in the American Psychiatric Association's *Diagnostic and Statistical Manual of Mental Disorders* (DSM-5) for major depressive disorder and has symptoms suggestive of generalized anxiety disorder and panic disorder. She is also having increasing difficulty with her day-to-day function and some memory changes, but within the context of anxiety. Although neuro-psychological testing might be warranted, there is not enough evidence to indicate a comorbid major neurocognitive disorder.

SCREENING TOOLS

There are several screening tools that can help to clarify the diagnosis of PTSD. The Primary Care PTSD Screen is a short screening tool in which the first question asks specifically for a history of trauma. If the answer is "no," then no further questions are asked and the screen is negative. If the response to this question is "yes," then the respondent is asked five additional yes/no questions. A positive screen (responding "yes" to three out of the five questions) requires further evaluation. The Impact of Events Scale–Revised is specifically targeted at older adults who have been exposed to any traumatic event. It consists of 22 questions with scores ranging from 0 to 88, with scores above 24 generally of concern. The PTSD CheckList–Civilian Version is a 17-item self-reported rating scale that has been validated in older adults. Scores range from 17 to 85 and may be interpreted based on the population being tested (lower cut-off for populations with higher prevalence rates, such as war veterans). A score of 50 and above is generally regarded as a positive screen regardless of the patient population.

The patient scored 25/30 on the Montreal Cognitive Assessment (MoCA). She displayed no problems with registration but had some difficulty with re-call. She had difficulty maintaining her attention and concentration during the evaluation. Her insight and judgment were limited. No visuospatial problems were noted on testing. She scored 55/85 on the PTSD CheckList. Results of lab tests were all within normal levels, and a computed tomography scan of the brain was also unremarkable.

PTSD IN OLDER ADULTS

Older adults may develop new-onset PTSD in later life or have a recurrence of previously remitted PTSD. Older adults often present with the same symptoms seen in younger adults. There have been a number of attempts to group symptoms by age, but no definitive conclusions have been reached at this time. In this case, the patient reported no prior history of PTSD and falls within the group of older adults who develop it in later life. Some researchers have hypothesized that exposure to trauma at different times in life could be protective against the development of PTSD. This is known as the *inoculation hypothesis*. On the other hand, repeated traumas could be cumulative and thus increase the risk of developing PTSD in later life, known as the *differential vulnerability hypothesis*. This may explain why populations that have been exposed to traumas stemming from racism, armed conflicts, or refugee status have higher reported rates of PTSD. The risk of PTSD in late life might also be related to changes in the primary role in an older adult's life as well as the increasing difficulty with day-to-day function that makes it more difficult to deal with memories of earlier traumas.

TREATMENT

Psychotherapy is the recommended first-line treatment modality for PTSD, with cognitive–behavioral therapy (CBT) being the preferred approach. Specific modalities of CBT for PTSD include exposure therapy (imagined, in vivo, or both), cognitive processing therapy (CPT), and Eye Movement Desensitization and Reprocessing (EMDR):

- *Exposure therapy* aims to help patients reduce symptoms and habituate by directly confronting their trauma repeatedly until they are able to gain control over their trauma-related memories and emotions. Older adults may have strong physiologic reactions to exposure therapy as a result of the increased prevalence of cardiovascular diseases, but this should not preclude the use of this therapeutic modality. Risks should be monitored closely and clearance from the appropriate specialist obtained if required.

- *CPT* uses CBT techniques to teach patients with PTSD how to evaluate, challenge, and change the distressing thoughts they have experienced that have been caused by their traumatic experiences. This process helps patients to reframe their understanding of their thoughts and in so doing change how they feel. CPT is usually done over a series of 12 sessions.

- In *EMDR*, patients bring up memories, images, emotions, and sensations of their trauma while their attention is engaged by a bilateral physical stimulus, such as repeated eye movements, looking at finger movements in front of their eyes, tapping, or music.

Psychoeducation is a reliably robust tool in the management PTSD in older patients as it provides them and their loved ones with information about the disorder, including its symptoms, course, treatment options, and potential outcomes.

Pharmacotherapy often plays a role in the management of PTSD when there are severe symptoms and/or comorbid psychiatric disorders, particularly ones that are not fully responsive to psychotherapeutic interventions (Table 16.2). As a starting point, the two selective serotonin reuptake inhibitors (SSRIs) sertraline and paroxetine have both been approved by the U.S. Food and Drug Administration (FDA) for PTSD. In older adults, sertraline would be the preferred choice due to its more tolerable side-effect profile and fewer drug–drug interactions. However, a variety of other antidepressants can be effective choices as well, especially as there is often comorbid anxiety and depression. Despite excellent efficacy, tricyclic antidepressants should generally be avoided in older individuals due to their cardiac and anticholinergic side effects as well as the nonlinear pharmacokinetics for most of the drugs in the class.

The use of benzodiazepines is not recommended in the management of PTSD at any age because they have the potential to aggravate dissociative symptoms, if present, and misuse is always a concern. In older adults, benzodiazepines carry additional risks, including increased risk of falls, confusion, and cognitive impairment. Select antipsychotics may be useful in patients with PTSD as well as with comorbid psychotic or mood disorders,

TABLE 16.2 **Medications and dosing strategies**

Drug	Dose range	Recommended titration schedule
Sertraline*	25–200 mg	Increase by 25 mg every 2–3 weeks
Paroxetine*	20–40 mg	Increase by 10 mg every 2–3 weeks
Escitalopram	5–20 mg	Increase by 5 mg every 2–3 weeks
Venlafaxine extended release	37.5–225 mg	Increase by 37.5–75 mg every 2–3 weeks
Mirtazapine	7.5–45 mg	Increase by 7.5 mg every 2–3 weeks
Quetiapine	25–600 mg	Increase by 25 mg in divided doses every 2–3 weeks
Prazosin	1–6 mg	Increase by 0.5–1 mg every 1–2 weeks

* FDA approved for treatment of PTSD

and have been studied as both monotherapy and augmentation. For example, one study of quetiapine found that doses that ranged between 50 mg and 800 mg and averaged between 200 and 300 mg were superior to placebo across PTSD symptom groups. Quetiapine may also be helpful in veterans with combat-related PTSD and with a history of traumatic brain injury. It is worth remembering, however, that antipsychotics carry increased risks of a variety of side effects, especially in older adults, not to mention the black box warning of potential cerebrovascular events and increased mortality in individuals with underlying dementia. Still, they are often used as augmentation agents for individuals with severe symptoms, including agitation, not responsive to baseline antidepressants. The key is judicious dosing and monitoring.

The alpha-1 antagonist prazosin has been shown to have some efficacy in the treatment of PTSD patients who have prominent re-experiencing symptoms such as nightmares. However, some more recent studies have suggested that the benefit may be no greater than with placebo.

This patient was trialed on multiple antidepressants (including sertraline and paroxetine), antipsychotics, and anxiolytics prior to, during, and after her hospitalization. She reported side effects with most of them and had little or no improvement with the rest. Her current medications were reviewed. She had been using an over-the-counter sleep aid that contained an antihistamine. This was discontinued due to the anticholinergic side effects of such medications. She was started on low-dose mirtazapine for her mood, anxiety, sleep, and appetite. However, at follow-up a month later she reported having side effects with mirtazapine, and it was discontinued as well. Other treatment modalities were discussed but were declined by the patient. At follow-up she was yet to start psychotherapy.

Unfortunately, older adults have been shown to have lower mental health service utilization than younger adults. There are also fewer programs that are specifically designed for them and their needs. In order to help older adults, like this patient, who would benefit from mental health services, it is important that clinicians develop ways to engage with them and their families resourcefully and efficiently to optimize engagement and to mitigate the risk that they will drop out of treatment.

KEY POINTS TO REMEMBER

- PTSD is a relatively common clinical condition in older adults and may be triggered by a wide range of traumas rather than just major events such as war, conflict, or assault.
- Careful screening and history-taking is the key to diagnosis. A range of screening instruments exist to help identify PTSD.
- Psychotherapy, especially CBT or approaches derived from it, represents the mainstay of treatment, although engagement in ongoing therapy can often be challenging, especially for older adults.
- Medications have an adjunctive role, primarily to manage significant mood or comorbid anxiety symptoms. SSRIs and antidepressants are considered the first-line agents for pharmacotherapy. Benzodiazepines should be avoided.

Further Reading

Averill PM, Beck JG. Posttraumatic stress disorder in older adults: A conceptual review. *J Anxiety Disord.* 2000;14(2):133–156.

Cook JM, Simiola V. Trauma and aging. *Curr Psychiatry Rep.* 2018;20(10):93.

Jakel R. Posttraumatic stress disorder in the elderly. *Psychiatr Clin North Am.* 2018;41(1):165–175.

Villarreal G, Hamner MB, Cañive JM, Robert S, Calais LA, Durklaski V, Zhai Y, Qualls C. Efficacy of quetiapine monotherapy in posttraumatic stress disorder: A randomized, placebo-controlled trial. *Am J Psychiatry.* 2016;173(12):1205–1212.

Mood Disorders

17 To switch or to augment: That is the question

Marie Anne Gebara and Jordan F. Karp

A 76-year-old woman is referred to psychiatry for symptoms of depression. She was euthymic until 2 years ago, when she experienced a mild heart attack. Two weeks later, her husband of 50 years died. She feels overwhelmed by taking care of her house and paying bills. She no longer enjoys seeing her grandchildren and worries that her memory is failing. She has periodic thoughts of taking an overdose of her oxycodone. However, she denies any intent or plan to actually kill herself. Her medical problems include hypertension, advanced osteoarthritis, and obstructive sleep apnea (OSA). She is having difficulty falling asleep and her appetite has waned over the past several months. A friend recommended she see a therapist, but she has not felt motivated. Her primary care physician treated her with sertraline 50 mg daily for nearly 6 weeks without any appreciable response, and then switched her to duloxetine 30 mg daily. She feels a little better but continues to feel sad and tired.

What do you do now?

In the diagnosis and management of late-life depression (LLD), one must ensure that the current treatment has been adequately implemented and must assess the risks of antidepressant exposure and age-specific conditions that may emerge or interact with these medications. One of the tenets of treating LLD is to "start low, go slow, but go all the way." This is because pharmacokinetic changes of aging include reductions in rates of absorption, changes in bioavailability, and an increase in the half-life of lipid-soluble drugs and the relative concentration for water-soluble drugs and metabolites. Medical comorbidities and polypharmacy increase the risk for pharmacokinetic and pharmacodynamic drug interactions. Clinicians must weigh the potentially serious adverse events associated with antidepressant use such as falls, hyponatremia, and gastrointestinal bleeding with both the relative safety of nonpharmacologic interventions and the risks inherent with untreated and/or undertreated depression.

Other treatment considerations include cardiac safety monitoring when prescribing tricyclic antidepressants (TCAs) and certain selective serotonin reuptake inhibitors (SSRIs). For example, in 2012 the U.S. Food and Drug Administration (FDA) issued a drug safety consideration for adults 60 and older to limit the maximum daily dose of the SSRI citalopram to 20 mg/day because of elevated risk of QTc prolongation. While still rare and not an absolute contraindication to prescribing, other adverse effects may occur more frequently in late life and require monitoring, such as serotonin syndrome, extrapyramidal side effects, and neuroleptic malignant syndrome.

As the patient's duloxetine is titrated, it would be appropriate to check her overall tolerance to the medication increase by asking about side effects and checking her sodium level.

An individualized risk-to-benefit analysis must be done for each patient, considering the potential risk of antidepressant use versus the risk of untreated depression, including increased psychiatric and other medical morbidity, all-cause mortality, quality of life, and suicide. In 2019 the American Geriatrics Society updated the Beers Criteria for potentially inappropriate medication use in older adults, cautioning against the use of antidepressants including SSRIs, serotonin–norepinephrine reuptake inhibitors (SNRIs), and TCAs based on fall risk. However, to this date, there have been no randomized controlled trials confirming the causal effect of these medications on falls in older adults. Therefore, while it is important to consider the guidelines to avoid potentially inappropriate medications in older adults, this must be done judiciously given the known risks of untreated depression in late life. Furthermore, several interventions can be implemented to mitigate fall risk in older adults, such as exercise programs, home safety interventions, and modification of footwear.

MEDICAL AND PSYCHIATRIC COMORBIDITIES

Medical and psychiatric comorbidities are more common in older patients and can affect both depression course and treatment outcomes. For example, any medical condition that causes pain, impairs physical ability, disrupts sleep, or impairs cognition can precipitate depressive symptoms, especially when these symptoms are chronic and require medications such as narcotics, steroids, muscle relaxants, or benzodiazepines that can further affect daily physical and mental function. Symptoms of anxiety are associated with more severe pathology and poorer treatment response. Substance use disorders, including alcohol and benzodiazepine use disorders, are highly comorbid with depression, and may worsen cognition, increase the risk of falls, and decrease the effectiveness of depression treatment. Any form for dementia can lessen the recognition of depressive symptoms and interfere with treatment response, especially when there is executive dysfunction.

Cognitive Status

Since age is the biggest risk factor for cognitive decline, an assessment of cognitive status is imperative. Depression is associated with cognitive decline and dementia; hence, treatment of depression is an effective approach to improve brain health. Cognitive impairment may develop after the onset of mood symptoms and is present in almost half of older patients with LLD. Even after the treatment of the mood symptoms, these impairments in domains such as executive function and processing speed often persist. Assessment of cognition can be done by surveying changes in function of instrumental activities of daily living such as medication management, finances, driving, and cooking. Additionally, screens of general cognitive function such as the Mini–Mental State Examination (MMSE) and the Montreal Cognitive Assessment (MoCA) can be used to identify changes and guide referral for comprehensive neuropsychological testing. With every patient, it is critical to identify and eliminate, if possible, medications that have brain toxicity, including benzodiazepines, narcotics, benzodiazepines, and other drugs with significant anticholinergic and antihistaminergic activity. When there are concerns about cognitive status, clinicians should evaluate the patient's ability to understand the risks, benefits, and alternative treatments as it relates to medication changes and side effects, and should involve surrogate decision-makers when indicated.

Fortunately, the patient scored 27/30 on her MoCA and has maintained independence in all of her instrumental activities of daily living, including driving, medication management, and finances. She was able to fully participate in all decisions regarding her treatment.

Pain

Pain and depression frequently co-occur in late life. Chronic pain predicts a slowed time to remission from depression. Therefore, screening for and ensuring optimal treatment of chronic pain may improve depression treatment outcomes.

Given the patient's osteoarthritis, her chronic knee pain may be considered an additive factor to her ongoing depression and she may be a good candidate for a referral to physical therapy in addition to non-opioid analgesic pharmacotherapy, intra-articular steroids or hyaluronic acid, or possibly referral for surgical evaluation.

Sleep

Depression is more challenging to treat in those with sleep disturbances, which can affect up to 35% of older adults. More specifically, around 85% of depressed older adults experience sleep disturbances, in the form of transient or chronic insomnia. Treating sleep disturbances can improve depression outcomes, but caution should be used when prescribing benzodiazepines and other sedative–hypnotics given the increased risk for falls, fractures, and cognitive impairment. Instead, physicians should provide education about appropriate sleep hygiene and consider more formal cognitive–behavioral therapy for insomnia, which has demonstrated good efficacy. OSA is common in older adults, is highly comorbid with LLD, and can interfere with antidepressant treatment response.

As it turns out, the patient had become noncompliant with her continuous positive airway pressure (CPAP) device as she felt that the mask was ill-fitting, and she felt too discouraged to put it on every night. She was able to get her mask refitted and noted improvement in both sleep and energy levels during the day.

ASSESSMENT

There are a variety of validated measures of depression severity. The Patient Health Questionnaire (PHQ-9) is a self-report screening questionnaire that can easily be administered to patients in the waiting room before their appointments. The scores range between 0 and 27, with higher scores indicating higher depression severity. Scores of 4 or less suggest minimal depression that may not need treatment, scores between 5 and 9 suggest mild to moderate depression, and scores that are 15 or higher suggest moderately severe to severe depression that requires treatment. Alternatively, the Geriatric Depression Scale (GDS) may also be used. It is a 30-item questionnaire with yes/no responses that surveys how patients have been feeling over the past week. There are both 15- and 5-item versions of the GDS. For individuals with dementia, the Cornell Scale for Depression in Dementia (CSDD) provides objectively observed items that patient and caregivers rate, with the score drawing from both. In its original form there are 19 items rated from 0 (absent) to 1 (mild or intermittent) and 2 (severe); scores >10 suggest probable depression and >18 indicate definite major depressive disorder.

Suicidal ideation is a symptom of depression and its presence may predict worse treatment outcomes and a more brittle response. Suicide attempts among older men have the highest success rate because they are often well planned and involve highly lethal means. Factors contributing to suicidal behavior include physical illness, grief and social isolation, alcohol abuse, hopelessness, anxiety, and a history of previous suicide attempt. A family history of completed or attempted suicide is also a risk factor for suicide. Standard clinical assessment includes asking about thoughts of death or dying and thoughts of self-harm. Clinicians should directly inquire about suicidal intent, plan, and access to lethal means such as firearms or medication stockpiles, and should mobilize family and sometime even law enforcement to remove them from the household. Patients who endorse suicidal ideation or passive death wishes but deny any intent should be asked about reasons for living and deterrents for suicide, such as religious beliefs or family. Suicide assessment tools such as the Suicidal Ideation Scale or the Columbia Suicide Severity Rating Scale can be administered in routine care for suicidal patients.

The patient denied any suicidal intent, and described her family and religion as main deterrents against suicide. She agreed to remove her late husband's firearm from her home.

TREATMENT STRATEGIES

Even though there is a tendency to reach first for antidepressant medication with older patients, it's always important to begin with supportive psychotherapeutic approaches and include formal psychotherapy when feasible. This is true even for individuals with mild to moderate cognitive impairment. Patients and families also need psychoeducation on the diagnosis and management of depression. Fortunately, there are effective nonpharmacologic alternatives to treating LLD, including cognitive–behavioral therapy (CBT), problem-solving therapy (PST), and interpersonal therapy (IPT). These are all manualized, time-limited therapies that have been shown to be effective in the treatment of LLD. Psychotherapy can be particularly helpful for patients with poor coping strategies, distorted thoughts and expectations, apathy, cognitive impairment, obsessive–compulsive features, and symptoms of anxiety and panic. It's also a critical adjunct to treatment when patients do not tolerate certain medication or combinations, or do not wish to add to their medication burden. Therapists should have training in working with older patients so they understand age-related factors and the role of common medical comorbidities.

The most efficacious approach to treating LLD with medications is to use treatment algorithms or decision trees that draw upon patient-specific demographic and clinical variables that help shape and predict treatment response. Favorable factors include early symptom improvement, lower baseline anxiety, and older age of onset, while negative predictors include a higher number of adequate antidepressant trials and sleep disturbances. An overall algorithm with recommended antidepressants in older adults is listed in Table 17.1.

TABLE 17.1 **Preferred antidepressants for LLD**

	Class	Preferred medications	Dose range (in mg)
First line	SSRIs	Sertraline	25–200
		Escitalopram	5–20
First line	SNRIs and similar agents	Duloxetine	60–120
		Venlafaxine	75–300
		Desvenlafaxine	50–100
		Mirtazapine	7.5–45
Second line (monotherapy or augmenting agent)	Serotonin agonists	Mirtazapine	7.5–45
Second line (monotherapy or augmenting agent)	Norepinephrine and dopamine reuptake inhibitors	Bupropion XL	150–450
Second line (augmenting agent)	Atypical antipsychotic	Aripiprazole	2–15
		Risperidone	0.25–1
		Quetiapine	25–150
Third line (augmenting agent)	Mood stabilizer	Lithium carbonate	150–600*
		Valproic acid	250–1,000
Third line	TCAs	Nortriptyline	50–100†

* Plasma level goal: 0.4–0.8 mmol/L; target 0.6mmol/L.
† Plasma level goal: 80–120 ng/mL.

First-line treatment with an SSRI such as escitalopram or sertraline is commonly accepted in practice. In Canada, concerns for QTc interval prolongation and torsades de pointes have led to a safety announcement recommending the limitation of escitalopram to 10 mg/day for adults over the age of 65. Fluoxetine is also an option but has a relatively long half-life, which can be problematic if there are side effects. It also tends to have more drug–drug interactions due to its inhibition of cytochrome 2D6. Paroxetine has been associated with anticholinergic side effects and tends to be more difficult to taper due to a greater risk of withdrawal effects. If a patient fails to respond to an SSRI, then the next step is to switch to an SNRIs such as venlafaxine, desvenlafaxine, or duloxetine. Mirtazapine boosts norepinephrine and serotonin selectively and is a preferred agent for individuals with insomnia and/or anorexia due to its common side-effect profile of sedation and appetite stimulation. Bupropion has a novel mechanism of action and appears to affect serotonin, norepinephrine, and dopamine, and is used often used in depressed patients with anergy or apathy due to its tendency to be more stimulating. Other newer antidepressants such as vortioxetine, vilazodone, and milnacipran are certainly viable choices, but there are fewer data about use in older individuals, especially those with cognitive impairment.

For partial responders to SSRIs and SNRIs, clinicians must first reassess the diagnosis and look for any comorbidities that are limiting response, such as pain, substance abuse, or cognitive impairment. Psychotherapeutic modalities should always be used. In terms of the medication trial, there are three options: (1) optimize the dose and ensure an adequate duration of 6 to 8 weeks; (2) switch to another antidepressant in the same or a different class; or (3) consider augmentation. A recent meta-analysis suggests that LLD may require a longer treatment trial (i.e., 10–12 weeks) as opposed to the recommended 4 to 6 weeks commonly cited with SSRI treatment.

When there is no treatment response on an adequate dose and duration, an different antidepressant should be used. It's often good to choose a different class of antidepressant, since prior SNRI trials are correlated with a lower likelihood of remission with another SNRI. Unfortunately, the number and type of past antidepressant trials appear to correlate inversely with the likelihood of response.

When there is some degree of response, augmentation is often the best route, especially since remission rates decline with increasing numbers of medication trials. Common augmentation strategies in older individuals include the addition of mirtazapine, bupropion, or an antipsychotic such as aripiprazole, risperidone, or quetiapine (while monitoring for common side effects of akathisia, parkinsonism, and sedation, respectively). Augmentation with either thyroid hormone (e.g., liothyronine or T3) or lithium carbonate is an option for individuals who either haven't responded to other augmentation or can't tolerate other strategies. Thyroid status must be assessed prior to the use of thyroid hormone, often in consultation with the patient's primary care physician or endocrinologist. Lithium must be used with extreme caution in older individuals due to its narrow safety range (which can easily be exceeded with commonly used medications such as nonsteroidal anti-inflammatory drugs [NSAIDs]) and effects on thyroid and renal function. Augmentation doses of lithium tend to be lower than those used to treat bipolar disorder, with blood levels used more to assess safety than efficacy. In general, augmentation strategies often yield clinical response in days to a week or two rather than in the many weeks required for full antidepressant response.

Despite the increase of duloxetine to 60 mg daily for 6 weeks, the patient's depression had only partially remitted, and she opted for augmentation with aripiprazole which was started at 2 mg daily and increased to 5 mg daily after 2 weeks. One month later, the patient's PHQ-9 score had dropped to 2, with her only complaints relating to minimal sleep disturbance and low energy.

For individuals who are complete nonresponders, it can take time to find the right combination of antidepressants or augmentation strategy, and there is the ongoing risk that comes with polypharmacy. The same strategies should be employed as with partial responders, with several options to consider. If first- and second-line treatments have failed, third-line treatments include switching to nortriptyline, which is the safest TCA in older adults as it carries the least risk of orthostatic hypotension and anticholinergic side effects. When prescribing a TCA, it is important to rule out any recent cardiovascular events, current orthostasis, or an electrocardiogram that shows preexisting cardiac conduction slowing such as first- or second-degree heart block, or QTc intervals >440 ms.

Treatment-resistant depression (TRD) is most commonly defined as the failure of two or more antidepressant trials of adequate dose and duration (which are subject to some debate). Based on the definition of failing at least two trials of antidepressants prescribed at the FDA-approved minimally therapeutic dose for adequate duration, more than half of depressed older adults qualify. TRD is associated with worse quality of life, disability, increase in death rates due to both suicide and all-cause mortality, worsened medical comorbidity, and cognitive decline and dementia. At this point, somatic treatments such as transcranial magnetic stimulation (TMS), electroconvulsive therapy (ECT) or ketamine (infusions or intranasal), can all be considered. Of the three, ECT has the best evidence of efficacy, and remains a relatively safe treatment option.

ONGOING MANAGEMENT

Close and frequent follow-up is essential, especially when starting a new treatment. This allows for ensuring compliance, monitoring for tolerability, providing reassurance about annoying but self-limiting side effects, psychoeducation, and ongoing supportive psychotherapy. It is helpful to engage caregivers in treatment planning as they are often reliable historians and may be able to detect depression response and relapse. They can also ensure treatment engagement and monitor and support medication compliance. It is also important to work across disciplines to include psychology, social work, rehabilitation specialists, and the patient's primary care physician. The implementation of a team approach helps to address co-occurring factors that contribute to depression such as falls and frailty, medical comorbidities (e.g., stroke, diabetes, pain, hypertension, OSA), and financial and legal stressors encountered by many older adults.

With the help of her primary care physician and physical therapist, the patient experienced meaningful improvement in the severity of both her OSA and osteoarthritis, contributing to further improvement in her depression.

KEY POINTS TO REMEMBER

- Ensure that the patient is receiving an adequate dose for an adequate amount of time before considering a medication change.
- Consider the patient's co-occurring medical and psychiatric comorbidities.
- Follow a treatment algorithm and measurement-based approach, but attend to patient- and age-specific conditions that may interfere with treatment response.
- Always include psychotherapeutic approaches, especially one of several time-limited and structured therapies that have shown efficacy in LLD.
- When prescribing antidepressant medications: "Start low, go slow, but go all the way."
- Augment for partial response and switch for nonresponse.
- Engage caregivers and implement a treatment team model.

Further Reading

Carley JA, Karp JF, Gentili A, Marcum ZA, Reid MC, Rodriguez E, Rossi MI, Shega J, Thielke S, Weiner DK. Deconstructing chronic low back pain in the older adult: Step-by-step evidence and expert-based recommendations for evaluation and treatment. Part IV: Depression. *Pain Med.* 2015;16(11):2098–2108.

Cristancho P, Lenard E, Lenze EJ, Miller JP, Brown PJ, Roose SP, Montes-Garcia C, Blumberger DM, Mulsant BH, Lavretsky H, Rollman BL, Reynolds CF 3rd, Karp JF. Optimizing Outcomes of Treatment-Resistant Depression in Older Adults (OPTIMUM): Study design and treatment characteristics of the first 396 participants randomized. *Am J Geriatr Psychiatry.* 2019;27(10):1138–1152.

Kok RM, Reynolds CF 3rd. Management of depression in older adults: A review. *JAMA.* 2017;317(20):2114–2122.

Mulsant BH, Blumberger DM, Ismail Z, Rabheru K, Rapoport MJ. A systematic approach to pharmacotherapy for geriatric major depression. *Clin Geriatr Med.* 2014;30(3):517–534.

Unutzer J, Park M. Older adults with severe, treatment-resistant depression. *JAMA.* 2012;308(9):909–918.

18 Expecting the expected

Susan W. Lehmann

An 82-year-old woman has a 50-year history of
bipolar I disorder. Over the years she has had
episodes of mania and of depression, but in
recent years she has had more depression. Her
last episode of severe depression was 6 years
ago, for which she was treated successfully
with electroconvulsive therapy (ECT). Over the
past 40 years 450mg of lithium daily has been
a mainstay of her pharmacologic management,
with normal serum creatinine levels. Her gait
has been steady and she has had a mild hand
tremor. In addition, she has been on nortriptyline
and risperidone. She was living independently
and at her most recent psychiatric follow-up,
she was not anxious and had no psychotic
symptoms. Her lithium level was 0.8 mEq/L
with normal renal function. She has a history of
mild hypercalcemia and concern about possible
hyperparathyroidism, but was told that there was
no need for medication treatment.

What do you do now?

This patient represents an unfortunately common clinical presentation for bipolar disorder in late life notable for clinical stability but with longer-term consequences of lithium therapy. Most mood-stabilizing medications require ongoing monitoring even in the face of stable blood levels and absence of clinical symptoms. The reasons for this are wide-ranging:

1. Aging-related changes in hepatic function may impact medications such as valproic acid or carbamazepine. Blood levels may slowly trend upwards. Simultaneously, blood levels that fall within the normal range may be too high for older adults and side effects such as tremor may manifest over time.

2. Aging-related changes in renal function may impact the blood level of medications such as lithium. As with hepatically metabolized mood stabilizers, blood levels that fall within the normal range may lead to side effects or even toxicity.

3. With age and long-term use, patients stabilized on second-generation antipsychotics may experience metabolic side effects such as weight gain, hypertension, and diabetes. Regular monitoring of blood levels for older adults on these medications is part of the standard of care.

4. Aging-related changes in body mass and drug metabolism impact the pharmacokinetics of most mood stabilizers. Thus, older adults may require lower doses than they did at younger ages. This must be counterbalanced with the risk of transient withdrawal or rebound symptoms during dose reduction, however, and should be done cautiously and supported by clear patient education about the process.

5. The principles of antidepressant management outlined in Chapter 17 apply to older adults with bipolar disorder who may be on long-term antidepressants as part of their medication regimen.

6. Increasing medical and psychiatric comorbidity is likelier to lead to polypharmacy as well as increased use of over-the-counter medications. For instance, medications such nonsteroidal anti-inflammatory drugs (NSAIDs), which affect renal function, or acetaminophen, which affects the

hepatic system, can significantly impact the metabolism of mood stabilizers and lead to toxicity, especially with lithium. Conversely, mood stabilizers and antidepressants can impact the efficacy of a range of other medications through inhibitory effects on the hepatic CYP450 system,

DETECTING AND MANAGING LONGER-TERM EFFECTS OF LITHIUM

This patient illustrates one of the concerns for clinicians who care for older patients treated chronically with lithium, especially for several well-established but not well-known adverse endocrinologic effects. Lithium-induced hypercalcemia is recognized by sustained serum calcium levels above the standard range (which is usually 8.5–10.5mg/dL); however, it is most accurately diagnosed by elevation of serum ionized calcium levels. Ionized calcium, which is about 40% of serum calcium, is physiologically active and is not bound to albumin or anions. Under usual circumstances, calcium is closely regulated by parathyroid hormone (PTH) secreted by the four parathyroid glands in the neck to prevent conditions of either hypocalcemia or hypercalcemia. Lithium is believed to alter the set-point of the calcium-sensing cells in the parathyroid glands. These cells normally respond to lower levels of calcium by secreting PTH, which then acts to decrease renal elimination of calcium by the kidneys, to increase calcium release from bones, and to increase absorption of calcium from the small intestine. When serum calcium levels are high, the calcium-sensing cells of the parathyroid glands suppress secretion of PTH, usually to below the lower reference limit. By altering the set-point, lithium changes the serum calcium level that stimulates the parathyroid glands to reduce PTH secretion. As a result, there is an increase in both serum total and ionized calcium without suppression of PTH release, leading to normal or high-normal levels of PTH. Lithium is also believed to have a direct effect on parathyroid cells to secrete PTH, which may contribute to development of hyperplasia and parathyroid adenomas causing secondary hyperparathyroidism.

Several risk factors for developing lithium-induced hypercalcemia and hyperparathyroidism include renal disease, female gender, and increased age. Patients with nephrogenic diabetes insipidus are more vulnerable to hypovolemia and dehydration, which can worsen hypercalcemia. Lithium-associated hyperparathyroidism has been noted to occur more frequently in women than men at a 3:1 incidence rate. The patient in question was at higher risk not only as an older female, but also due to her chronic diabetes mellitus, which is a cause of small-vessel vascular disease and renal function impairment, even though her serum creatinine was in the normal range. Interestingly, while older patients may be more vulnerable to developing lithium-associated hypercalcemia and hyperparathyroidism due to concomitant renal disease or vitamin D deficiency, duration of lithium treatment has not been identified as a risk factor. In fact, cases of hypercalcemia and hyperparathyroidism have been reported in patients treated with lithium for durations of time ranging from 1 month to 30 years.

Lithium-induced hyperparathyroidism is a type of secondary hyperparathyroidism and differs from primary hyperthyroidism in a number of ways. Most notably, in lithium-induced hyperparathyroidism there is hypocalciuria, normal serum phosphate levels, and elevated serum magnesium levels. This is in contrast to primary hyperparathyroidism, which is characterized by hypercalciuria, low serum phosphate levels, and mildly elevated serum magnesium level (Table 18.1). The clinical picture of primary hyperparathyroidism includes nephrolithiasis, bone resorption, mental status changes, and pancreatitis or peptic ulcer disease. In contrast, lithium-induced hyperparathyroidism is often asymptomatic.

TABLE 18.1 **Lithium-associated hyperparathyroidism compared with primary hyperparathyroidism**

	Lithium-associated hyperparathyroidism	Primary hyperparathyroidism
Serum calcium	Elevated	Elevated
Serum phosphate	Normal	Low
Urinary calcium	Hypocalciuria	Hypercalciuria
Serum magnesium	Elevated	Slightly elevated
Renal cyclic AMP	Low-normal	High

However, lithium-associated hypercalcemia and hyperparathyroidism can cause symptoms such as weakness and fatigue, constipation, bone pain, or abdominal pain. Patients treated with lithium who develop hypercalcemia have been reported to be at increased risk for cardiac conduction abnormalities. In addition, elevation in serum calcium due to lithium can be a precipitant or underlying cause for delirium, confusion, or cognitive impairment. In rare instances, lithium-associated hyperparathyroidism has caused psychotic symptoms, including paranoia and hallucinations. For these reasons, it is important to monitor patients for elevation in calcium levels and to follow up with assessment of PTH and ionized calcium levels if screening serum calcium levels become elevated, even if patients appear asymptomatic. Patients who present with possible lithium-induced hypercalcemia/hyperparathyroidism should be referred to an endocrinologist, who may decide to treat the patient with cinacalcet to lower calcium levels to the normal range. Occasionally, patients may need surgical evaluation if a parathyroid adenoma is detected. Significantly, as with hypothyroidism due to lithium treatment, it is usually not necessary to discontinue lithium treatment if calcium can be normalized by treatment with cinacalcet. This is especially important for patients for whom lithium is a key part of their medication regimen for mood stability.

Current national and international guidelines for management of bipolar disorder include recommendation to screen patients on lithium regularly for thyroid disease and for renal effects of lithium treatment. At present, there are no specific guidelines for screening for hypercalcemia or hyperparathyroidism due to lithium treatment. Given that older patients on lithium therapy may be at greater risk, especially if they have comorbid renal disease, it is prudent to screen all older patients for hypercalcemia. It is recommended that serum calcium levels be checked yearly. If screening serum calcium levels are elevated, further testing should include ionized calcium and PTH levels and referral to an endocrinologist for further evaluation.

The patient was referred to an endocrinologist, who found that she had an elevated PTH of 103 pg/mL and confirmed the diagnosis of lithium-associated hyperparathyroidism. While she remained asymptomatic in terms of somatic manifestations, her endocrinologist started her on cinacalcet at a dose of 30 mg daily, which was effective in lowering her serum calcium a month later to 10.4, in the normal range. Given that lithium was felt to be essential to treating her bipolar disorder, it was continued and lithium serum levels remained at 0.7 mEq/L, with continued mood well-being.

KEY POINTS TO REMEMBER

- The primary principle of managing bipolar disorder in late life involves careful oversight of mood stabilizers and antidepressants. Clinicians must monitor clinical symptoms, toxicity, blood levels of medications as appropriate, and the potential for emergence of long-term side effects.
- Lithium-induced hypercalcemia and lithium-associated hyperparathyroidism may develop at any time with lithium treatment, but older adults with renal and vascular impairment may be more vulnerable.
- Lithium-induced hypercalcemia is diagnosed by sustained elevation of serum calcium levels above the reference range and is believed to occur as a direct effect of lithium altering the set-point of the calcium-sensing cells of the parathyroid glands.
- Endocrinology referral should be done and treatment may require cinacalcet, but lithium treatment can usually continue for patients who are responsive to lithium and are benefiting from lithium treatment for their mood disorder.

Further Reading

Lehmann SW, Lee J. Lithium-associated hypercalcemia and hyperparathyroidism in the elderly: What do we know? *J Affect Disord.* 2013;146(2):151–157.

Livingston C, Rampes H. Lithium: A review of its metabolic adverse effects. *J Psychopharmacol.* 2006;20(3):347–355.

McHenry CR, Lee K. Lithium therapy and disorders of the parathyroid glands. *Endocr Pract.* 1996;2(2):103–109.

McNight RF, Adida M, Budge K, Stockton S, Goodwin GM, Geddes JR. Lithium toxicity profile: A systematic review and meta-analysis. *Lancet.* 2012;379:721–728.

Moe SM. Disorders involving calcium, phosphorus, and magnesium. *Prim Care.* 2008;35(2):215–337.

19 Life is not worth living

Ali Asghar-Ali and Richa Lavingia

A 75-year-old man with a history of congestive heart failure, arthritis, and diabetes presents for a follow-up appointment. You have been managing his chronic pain and medical comorbidities for the past year. Over the past few months, he has reported worsening hip and back pain that is restricting his walking. He seems more irritable. At his last appointment 2 weeks ago, he reported that he had not talked with friends or family for days and had started drinking daily. Today, he voices frustrations about ongoing pain despite trying several pharmacologic and nonpharmacologic interventions. He states that he has been feeling like "life is not worth living anymore". While he had reported sadness after the death of his wife 3 months ago, he had never expressed suicidal thoughts. He reports feeling depressed for a few months, and that the chronic pain and loss of his wife have made him want to end his life. He reveals that he has been thinking about shooting himself and has been keeping a loaded gun on his bedside table.

What do you do now?

Older adults in the United States, particularly older White men, are at high risk of attempting and completing suicide. As the number of older adults continues to increase, geriatric suicide will remain a significant public health concern. The most common method of suicide among older adults is the use of firearms, followed by poisoning. In 2017, adults aged 85 years and older had a suicide rate of 20.1 per 100,000 individuals, second only to those aged 45 to 54 years (20.2 per 100,000). Among men, those 65 years and older had the highest suicide rate of any age group (31.0 per 100,000, compared to 5.0 per 100,000 among women aged 65 years and older). Over the past decade the suicide rate has increased for older adults in all age groups. Suicide attempts made by older adults are more likely to result in death than those made by younger adults, possibly due in part to their greater frailty and the use of more lethal means of suicide, such as firearms. Rates of suicide in nursing homes and assisted living facilities do not need to be reported by federal authorities. However, at least by some estimates, rates of older adult suicide in nursing homes and assisted living mirror their community-dwelling counterparts.

EVALUATION OF RISK

Suicide is a complex and multifactorial issue that involves a longitudinal interplay among risk factors, protective factors, and personality traits. The suicide evaluation and plan should include identification of risk factors and protective factors; inquiry about suicidal thoughts, plan, intent to die by suicide, past attempts, and self-injurious behaviors; assessment of risk and appropriate intervention; and, finally, documentation of the patient's level of risk for suicide, recommended intervention, and rationale for both.

In this case, significant risk factors for suicide include the patient's male sex, chronic pain with recent worsening, functional impairment, medical comorbidities, social isolation after the loss of his wife, daily alcohol use, and access to lethal means. Other important risk factors for suicide in older adults include psychiatric disorders, history of prior suicide attempts, and neurocognitive disorders (see Table 19.1 for a list of selected risk factors and management strategies).

The presence of a psychiatric illness, in particular major depressive disorder (MDD) and bipolar disorder, is a significant risk factor for attempted and completed suicide. Clinicians should keep in mind that depression in older adults can manifest with sadness or tearfulness, irritability, retreating from social situations, anhedonia, and lack of interest.

Substance use is also a risk factor. In this patient, heavy alcohol consumption increases his risk for suicide. Alcohol use disorder has been linked to suicidal behavior, though delineating the relationship between the two is complicated by the presence of other psychiatric disorders and sociodemographic risk factors. Rates of opioid misuse and abuse have also increased significantly over the past two decades, as has the number of suicides involving opioids. Patients with chronic pain and a co-occurring psychiatric disorder who are prescribed opioids are at increased risk of opioid use disorder and should be closely monitored.

As a group, older adults are particularly affected by physical illness and polypharmacy. Specific medical conditions, such as malignancy, seizure disorders, and HIV, are associated with increased rates of suicide. Of note, the greater the number of physical illnesses, the greater the risk for suicide in older adults. Perceived health status likely influences risk as well, though the evidence is limited.

Older adults are also much more prone to functional impairment, major neurocognitive disorder/dementia, and other forms of disability than younger adults. Functional impairment, whether from physical or cognitive limitations, can lead to frustration and depression among older adults, as well as the sense that they pose a burden to their loved ones or to society in general. This feeling of burdensomeness can heighten an older adult's suicide risk. Neurocognitive impairment, including frontal executive dysfunction and dementia, has also been associated with a higher risk of suicide, and risk is heightened in those who have also been treated for psychiatric disorders. The period following a diagnosis of dementia may represent a time of elevated suicide risk.

Finally, stressful life events and social isolation can elevate an older adult's suicide risk. Psychosocial stressors can include financial stress, conflict in relationships, grief and bereavement after a loss, and difficult life transitions, such as the loss of independence after moving to a nursing home. Social isolation, which can be a result of the loss of social support and loved ones, lack of participation in community activities, or living alone, is also associated with increased risk of suicide.

TABLE 19.1   Selected risk factors for suicide and management strategies in older adults

Risk factor	Strategy/intervention
Psychiatric illness (e.g., MDD, substance use disorder)	· Biological interventions: pharmacotherapy (e.g., selective serotonin reuptake inhibitors [SSRIs], serotonin–norepinephrine reuptake inhibitors [SNRIs]), electroconvulsive therapy (ECT), transcranial magnetic stimulation (TMS) · Psychotherapy: cognitive–behavioral therapy (CBT), dialectical behavioral therapy, problem-solving therapy · Psychosocial: remove substances from the home; substance use treatment
Access to firearms or other lethal means	· Request to remove firearms and old or unused medications · Encourage securing firearms and medication storage options (gun safe, gun lock, medication lockbox) · Limit prescription quantities when possible
Functional impairment/ disability and limited mobility	· Encourage resumption of previously enjoyed activities with modifications (e.g., making video calls with friends and family if unable to visit in person) · Psychotherapy: CBT, problem-solving therapy
Social isolation/lack of meaning in life	· Psychotherapy: CBT, problem-solving therapy · Psychosocial: Encourage participation in hobbies, volunteering, community activities, local senior centers, and support groups

In addition to risk factors, clinicians should consider personality traits and protective factors. Personality traits that predispose to suicide include rigidity, neuroticism, and impulsivity. Protective factors include religion and spirituality, social connectedness, effective coping strategies, access to care for physical and mental health conditions, and a sense of meaning and purpose in life. Identifying protective factors allows clinicians to approach suicide prevention from a strengths-based perspective and mobilize resources that will enhance the safety of their patients.

SCREENING

Given the complex nature of suicide, there are several diagnostic and therapeutic modalities to consider. First, because MDD is a key risk factor, primary care clinicians can implement screening procedures to detect older adults with depressive symptoms. Late-life depression is often undiagnosed and untreated, and the majority of treatment for late-life depression occurs in the primary care setting. Evidence is limited on the effectiveness of universal screening for depression and suicidality, but clinicians can consider screening those at risk, such as those with medical comorbidities, functional impairment, history of psychiatric illness or suicide attempt, or recent psychosocial stressors, and all adults aged 85 years and older. Several validated screening tools have been developed for use with older adults, including the Geriatric Depression Scale (GDS) and its shortened version, the GDS-S.

Clinicians can also use general screening tools, such as the Patient Health Questionnaire-9 (PHQ-9). Item 9 on the PHQ-9, which assesses suicidal ideation, has been predictive of completed suicide in some studies of older adults. However, these tools are not perfectly sensitive and should be considered in the context of a comprehensive evaluation. Other screening options include clinician-administered scales, such as the Cornell Scale for Depression in Dementia (CSDD), the Hamilton Depression Rating Scale (HAM-D), and the Columbia Suicide Severity Rating Scale (C-SSRS). The CSDD is specifically designed for older adults with dementia. It measures mood and ideational disturbances, cyclic functions, behavioral disturbances, and physical signs, such as loss of appetite. The HAM-D is a general assessment of depression, but there is limited evidence on its validity with older adults.

The C-SSRS is a validated scale that assesses suicidal ideation and behaviors. There are several versions of the scale available, including a lifetime/recent scale and a shortened screener scale. Clinicians can also administer the Risk Assessment Page, which measures risk factors and protective factors, in conjunction with the C-SSRS. Though not validated specifically for older adults, the C-SSRS has been used in this population.

STEPS AFTER IDENTIFYING SUICIDALITY

If a patient endorses suicidal thoughts, the clinician should evaluate the acuity and severity of suicide risk, identify an appropriate intervention, and document the rationale behind the risk-level determination and intervention. Those who report suicidal ideation with a plan and intent to die by suicide and appear unable to maintain their safety at home generally require direct observation to maintain safety pending rapid psychiatric hospitalization.

The patient was hospitalized for 7 days and scheduled for a follow-up appointment 4 days after his discharge. During his hospitalization, he was started on a low dose of a selective serotonin reuptake inhibitor, participated in group psychotherapy, and met with a substance abuse counselor. The team also communicated closely with his children, who, with the patient's permission, removed his gun and alcohol from his home. Prior to discharge, his psychiatrist worked with him and his family to create a safety plan and arrange follow-up visits for psychotherapy and medication management. His pain was addressed with a consult to the pain management team, which he found helpful. The team also identified patient strengths, such as his strong family support, long history of volunteering at church, and financial stability.

COLLABORATIVE SAFETY PLANNING

Patients at lower risk, such as those with suicidal ideation but no specific intent, plan, or preparatory behaviors, can be cared for in the outpatient setting. For individuals with an underlying psychiatric illness or psychosocial stressors, treatment may include pharmacotherapy, psychotherapy, social interventions, and specialty psychiatric care, as needed. Other modifiable risk factors, such as social isolation and access to lethal means, should be addressed routinely.

Clinicians can work with patients to mitigate suicide risk by using a collaborative safety planning model. There are several types of crisis response plans and safety plans. Here is one systematic, six-step process.

Step 1

The clinician and patient should consider warning signs for suicidality, including physical signs, such as insomnia; changes in mood and thoughts, such as hopelessness and cravings for substances; and behaviors, such as self-isolation. Through this step, the patient can gain a better understanding of circumstances that increase risk for suicide and may require mitigating strategies.

Step 2

The clinician and patient should discuss internal coping strategies that the patient may employ in the face of suicidal thoughts, such as guided meditation, reading, taking a walk, and paying attention to sleep. Patients with functional impairment that limits particular activities should be encouraged to identify alternate activities or to participate in modified versions of activities they enjoy. For example, a patient who can no longer read print may be able to listen to an audiobook.

Steps 3 to 5

The emphasis is on the importance of social connectedness, identifying friends and family members who support the patient, and connecting the patient to community resources and agencies. Community resources, such as senior centers, may help older adults who are socially isolated. Depending on the patient's health status and risk factors, referral to other community agencies may be warranted. For example, a patient with a recent diagnosis of Parkinson's disease might be referred to the Parkinson's Foundation.

Step 6

The clinician and patient should discuss ways to make the home environment safer. Patients should be asked about firearms in the home. If possible, firearms should be removed. If the patient is unwilling to remove the firearms, other options can be discussed, such as the use of a gun safe or gun lock, as well as separate storage of unloaded firearms and ammunition. Other items that may need to be removed from the home include alcohol and other substances, poisons, and expired and unused medications.

As part of this step, the clinician should also ask the patient to identify things that give their life meaning and make life worth living and to write these in the safety plan. The safety plan should be readily accessible to the patient. It can either be written as a document for the patient to carry, with copies given to friends and family members if the patient agrees, or it can be entered on a safety plan application on the patient's mobile device.

During the safety planning process with older adults, clinicians should make accommodations for functional impairments, if present. These may include incorporating hearing devices such as a pocket talker, which can reduce background noise and amplify sounds, allowing older adults to better hear and participate in conversations. Other strategies include speaking slowly, repeating information, and providing written information for the patient's reference. If the patient is comfortable with this, a family member or friend should be included in the development of the plan. Patients with cognitive impairment may need a simplified plan and the necessary involvement of family, friends, or caregivers.

Clinicians working with older adults at risk for suicide should remember that suicide can occur in a variety of settings, including nursing homes and assisted living facilities. Evaluating the safety of the environment in these settings is important, and the same precautions should be taken in terms of removing possible means of suicide. When possible, and when the patient gives permission, the clinician can communicate and share the safety plan with staff and caregivers.

KEY POINTS TO REMEMBER

- Older adults are at high risk of attempting and completing suicide, particularly those with psychiatric illnesses, multiple medical comorbidities, previous suicide attempts, functional impairment, recent psychosocial stressors, and social isolation.
- When assessing suicidality, clinicians should identify risk and protective factors; ask about suicidal ideation, past attempts, suicide plans, and intent to complete suicide; determine the patient's suicide risk level and appropriate intervention; and document the rationale for this determination.
- Suicide safety planning should involve a systematic, collaborative approach.

Further Reading

Conejero I, Olié E, Courter P, Calati R. Suicide in older adults: Current perspectives. *Clin Interv Aging*. 2018;13:691–699.

Heisel MJ, Neufeld E, Flett GL. Reasons for living, meaning in life, and suicide ideation: Investigating the roles of key positive psychological factors in reducing suicide risk in community-residing older adults. *Aging Mental Health*. 2016;20(2):195–207.

Mezuk B, Lohman M, Leslie M, Powell V. Suicide risk in nursing homes and assisted living facilities: 2003–2011. *Am J Public Health*. 2015;105(7):1495–1502.

Okolie C, Dennis M, Thomas S, John A. A systematic review of interventions to prevent suicidal behaviors and reduce suicidal ideation in older people. *Int Psychogeriatrics*. 2017;29(11):1801–1824.

Seyfried LS, Kales HC, Ignacio RV, Conwell Y, Valenstein M. Predictors of suicide in patients with dementia. *Alzheimers Dementia*. 2011;7(6):567–573.

Stanley B, Brown GK. Safety planning intervention: A brief intervention to mitigate suicide risk. *Cogn Behav Practice*. 2012;19(2):256–264.

Substance Abuse and Mental Health Services Administration (SAMHSA). SAFE-T: Suicide Assessment Five-Step Evaluation and Triage for mental health professionals. https://www.integration.samhsa.gov/images/res/SAFE_T.pdf

20 Withering away

Mario Fahed and Kristina Zdanys

An 83-year-old man is brought to the emergency department, by his spouse after several months of changes in his mood and behavior. He makes poor eye contact, and his speech is slow and sporadic. His spouse reveals that he has become increasingly passive and has stopped participating in activities that he used to enjoy. He has lost more than 10% of his body weight over 4 months. He is drowsy and but he denies suicidal ideation and does not express delusional thoughts. His spouse shares that he lost some of his retirement savings to a phone scam, but they remain financially secure. He has fallen twice in the past 2 months while getting out of bed and has not showered in weeks. He has had recurrent depressive episodes but without hospitalizations. There is no history of mania or substance abuse. He appears medically stable. He was a former banker, and after retirement he spent his days with his friends, but has not engaged with them for months.

What do you do now?

This case demonstrates several complex diagnostic dilemmas. On the one hand, the patient has symptoms that meet criteria for a severe, recurrent major depressive disorder. There is also clear neurocognitive impairment and functional decline that may be associated in part with the depression, but appears to exceed the severity that may be expected from depression alone. His frail physical presentation raises concern for additional underlying medical conditions, although initial work-up in the emergency department did not uncover any acute illness necessitating a medical admission. Although the patient is not suicidal and does not pose a danger to others, he does seem gravely disabled to the point of possibly needing inpatient psychiatric hospitalization.

Put together, a new diagnostic entity emerges in this case: failure to thrive (FTT). Both FTT and frailty are multifactorial geriatric syndromes, meaning they are conditions that do not fit into any one disease category. Characteristics of these syndromes are listed in Boxes 20.1 and 20.2. It is sometimes difficult to ascertain whether depressive symptoms preceded or resulted from FTT, and this relationship may be bidirectional. Experts have come to agree on three components whose interaction results in FTT: frailty, disability, and neuropsychiatric impairment.

ASSESSMENT

Although the patient's medical work-up in the emergency department did not yield any results that would necessitate a medical admission, a more in-depth medical work-up should be performed while the patient is on the inpatient psychiatric unit. It is important to obtain a full review of systems that is both constitutional (e.g., fever, night sweats) and organ-focused. Regarding his weight loss, possible underlying malignancy should be ruled out. Other contributing factors associated with weight loss may include loss of olfaction (thus affecting sense of taste), dry mouth from medications, or poor dentition. Assessments for dysphagia (including a swallow evaluation), availability of nutrition in the home (secondary to economic or logistical impediments), and a physical therapy assessment would also be indicated to determine his fall risk and level of observation required at the time of admission.

Additional laboratory work-up, if not already completed in the emergency department, would include a urinalysis, complete blood count with differential, complete metabolic panel including hepatic function, lipid panel, and levels of magnesium, vitamin D, calcium, phosphate, thyroid stimulating hormone (TSH), and vitamin B_{12}. Measurement of C-reactive protein (CRP) and erythrocyte sedimentation rate (ESR) may be useful if there is suspicion for malignancy or inflammatory disease. HIV and syphilis testing may also be ordered as appropriate. To evaluate for potential malignancy, a fecal occult blood test and chest X-ray may be helpful. Brain imaging such as non-contrast computed tomography (CT) of the head may rule out acute cerebrovascular injury, and magnetic resonance imaging (MRI) can provide a more detailed picture of chronic microvascular changes that often contribute to changes in mood, behavior, and cognition.

Clinicians should obtain a careful timeline of symptom emergence to delineate between hypoactive delirium (acute onset, with waxing-and-waning attention and sensorium), depression (subacute onset over weeks to months with associated anhedonia, depressed mood, and somatic complaints), and dementia (protracted onset that is either gradual or stepwise, with deficits in other cognitive domains and associated functional impairment). It is important to perform a baseline cognitive screen on admission. Though the score may be impacted by the neurocognitive impairment of depression, it often helps to track improvement in cognitive scores as antidepressants are started and to repeat this screen after remission of depressive symptoms to assess for underlying cognitive impairment. The patient in question may not be able to engage in a full neuropsychological battery during hospitalization given the severity of his depressive symptoms, but if available he may benefit from initial consultation with a neuropsychologist on the inpatient unit, with a plan to undergo full testing when his depressive symptoms improve.

It is important to assess the role of psychosocial factors in the patient's presentation, including those that may contribute negatively to the patient's present condition and those that may help ease the patient's symptoms or provide support when the patient is discharged from the hospital. Psychosocial factors may or may not be modifiable. Considerations include risk of abuse, substance use, availability of family and community supports, access to care and caregivers, financial resources, availability of transportation, and physical accessibility of the home environment.

TREATMENT

The treatment of FTT should always be managed by a multidisciplinary team, given all of the comorbid factors that need attention simultaneously. At the same time, there needs to be the central leadership of both an internist and a psychiatrist to expeditiously manage the case, since time is of the essence. Even a few days and certainly a few weeks of poor hydration and nutrition and overall deconditioning can have dire consequences in someone who is already compromised. The geriatric psychiatrist will be key in establishing and clarifying the differential diagnosis and then providing critical therapeutic and pharmacologic interventions. In many cases, he or she will also serve as the team leader along with the geriatric internist. The other team members and their various roles are outlined in Table 20.1, although additional consultations certainly may be indicated.

TABLE 20.1 Roles on the multidisciplinary team

Team member	Role
Team leader (geriatric internist or psychiatrist)	· Coordinate all diagnostic procedures and decision-making about the treatment plan · Serve as liaison with patient and family/surrogates · Be aware of all findings about the patient and disseminate them to key team members
Geriatric internist	· Assess medical diagnoses and degree of frailty · Assist with management of comorbid medical conditions · Play key role in decision-making · May provide pre-procedure clearance if ECT is considered
Nursing staff	· Monitor pain · Monitor vital signs · Monitor food intake · Administer medications
Social worker	· Assess psychosocial factors impacting care · Discharge planning (services, level of care)
Neuropsychologist	· Assess neurocognitive status via cognitive screens and appropriate neuropsychological tests · Advise team on appropriate expectations given baseline neurocognitive abilities · Provide appropriate psychotherapeutic support
Occupational therapist	· Assess activities of daily living and safety · Provide appropriate therapy
Physical therapist	· Assess strength, ambulation, and fall risk · Provide therapy for mobilization, strength, coordination and balance to mitigate deconditioning and fall risk
Pharmacist	· Consult for polypharmacy · Evaluate potential medication interactions and side effects contributing to presentation
Speech therapist	· Assess swallow function · Provide speech therapy, as needed
Nutritionist	· Assess nutritional needs · Accommodate changes in food consistency based on swallow evaluation · Consider dietary supplements for increasing caloric intake

Pharmacologic approaches for FTT follow the same basic principles as in other geriatric prescribing: Begin at a low dose and titrate to the lowest effective dose, which may be equivalent to a full dose used in younger adults if tolerated and required. Polypharmacy should be minimized. Benzodiazepines, tricyclic antidepressants, and other potentially inappropriate medications with high risk of side effects in older adults should be avoided, if possible. Risk of interaction with the patient's other medications should be considered.

It is important to understand why a particular medication is chosen. Antidepressants treat depression, which is a component of FTT, and in treating depression the overall FTT syndrome may improve. But it would be misleading to say that antidepressants treat FTT directly. Similarly, if it is determined that a chronic illness is contributing to the symptoms of FTT, treatment of that underlying illness may then result in improvement of FTT.

Mirtazapine is a useful medication for patients who present with FTT. In addition to its antidepressant effects it is also helpful in improving appetite and promoting weight gain, which will help a patient with FTT regardless of the degree of depression in the presentation. Mirtazapine is highly sedating, which is a benefit for patients experiencing sleep disturbance; however, for this patient, who is quite lethargic, it would be important to note whether daytime grogginess worsened after starting mirtazapine. As with almost all antidepressants, mirtazapine may also increase risk of falls. A starting dose among older adults can be as low as 3.75 mg at bedtime, though a target treatment dose of 15 to 45 mg may be needed for good effect. With FTT with more severe states of depression, augmentation of mirtazapine could be considered with selective serotonin reuptake inhibitors (SSRIs) or serotonin–norepinephrine reuptake inhibitors (SNRIs). A classic treatment approach for severe depression in older adults is the combination of mirtazapine and venlafaxine. Less commonly used pharmacologic approaches that could be considered in FTT among older adults include appetite stimulants such as cyproheptadine or dronabinol.

Electroconvulsive therapy (ECT) is a fast, effective, and overall safe treatment option for older adults with severe depression coupled with life-threatening FTT, such as when there is refusal to eat or take critical medications or other treatments. It is also indicated with FTT associated with treatment-resistant depression, catatonia, and/or psychosis.

The patient's lab studies showed low albumin and normalization of BUN and creatinine after hydration. The dietary team recommended starting supplement shakes once daily. The swallow evaluation did not show any dysphagia. The physical therapist recommended shower ramps without any assistive devices, and engaged the patient 4 days per week in strengthening exercises, which he did with some reluctance. The occupational therapist was unable to assess him due to lack of cooperation with the evaluation. He responded "I don't know" to most of the prompts during the cognitive screening assessment, a pattern usually seen in depression. He was started on mirtazapine 7.5 mg at night, which was increased to 15 mg three nights later. He tolerated mirtazapine without any adverse effects. After 1 week, he spent fewer than 2 hours in bed during the daytime and became more engaged socially and in unit activities. After 2 weeks, he consistently was eating greater than 75% of his meals and had gained 5 pounds. At no point did he demonstrate delusional thinking or express suicidal thoughts. He was discharged to home with a visiting nurse and in-home physical therapy, with the plan to follow up for psychiatric care at an outpatient clinic.

Although it is encouraging that the patient demonstrated improvement in appetite, weight, energy, and activity level on the inpatient psychiatric unit, close outpatient follow-up is imperative. Perhaps most intrinsic to a successful outpatient treatment is that the psychiatrist establishes a positive rapport with the patient and the patient's main caregivers and everyone works together as a team. Once a patient recovers from FTT, there remains a need for ongoing long-term attention and rehabilitation.

KEY POINTS TO REMEMBER

- Failure to thrive (FTT) is a multifactorial geriatric syndrome characterized by weight loss, decreased appetite, poor nutrition, dehydration, depressive symptoms, inactivity, impaired immune function and low cholesterol.
- The relationship of FTT and depression may be bidirectional, and comorbid dementia is common.

- The work-up of FTT should consider factors such as medical illness, hypoactive delirium, neurocognitive disorder, and psychosocial stressors in addition to depression. Much of the medical work-up will look for factors that could be causing weight loss, including issues relating to dentition, chewing, swallowing, nutrition and underlying malignancy.
- Treatment of depression may improve FTT, and antidepressants such as mirtazapine as well as ECT should be considered.

Further Reading

Katz IR, DiFilippo S. Neuropsychiatric aspects of failure to thrive in late life. *Clin Geriatr Med*. 1997;13(4):623–638.

Robertson RG, Montagnini M. Geriatric failure to thrive. *Am Fam Physician*. 2004;70(2):343–350.

Rocchiccioli JT, Sanford JT. Revisiting geriatric failure to thrive: A complex and compelling clinical condition. *J Gerontol Nurs*. 2009;35(1):18–24.

Verdery RB. Clinical evaluation of failure to thrive in older people. *Clin Geriatr Med*. 1997;13(4):769–778.

Sad or just unconcerned?

Jennifer Junko Holiman, Kathryn Kieran, and Caroline S. Bader

A 85-year-old woman who lives by herself is referred for evaluation by her primary care doctor for symptoms of depression with prominent lack of motivation. She has a diagnosis of Parkinson's disease with associated mild dementia, and with minimal response to carbidopa/levodopa. For the past 6 months she has shown decreased interest in spending time with her family. She rarely initiates tasks at home or conversations. She was strangely unconcerned when one of her grandchildren was injured in a car accident. In general she is calm and placid and denies emotional distress. A recent medical work-up was unremarkable, and an magnetic resonance imaging (MRI) of her brain showed mild atrophy with hippocampal shrinkage and slightly widened ventricles, similar to a scan 5 years prior. She denies feeling depressed, nervous, or upset but her friends and family are concerned about the change in her overall demeanor. There were no thoughts of hopelessness or worthlessness, or any suicidal thoughts. Lab tests were normal.

What do you do now?

Apathy and depression can often be quite difficult to distinguish from one another, particularly in the context of a neurocognitive disorder such as Alzheimer's disease (AD). Apathy is a withdrawal of activity without mood change, while depression by definition must be accompanied by a change in mood, often with guilt, which is sometimes verbally expressed as being a "bad" or unworthy person. Apathy will often present as a lack of interest in usual activities or social engagements, and a loss of emotional engagement with reduced affect. In contrast, depression will specifically include low mood and voicing of feeling sad, helpless, or hopeless. While both apathy and depression are frequently present in neurocognitive disorders, apathy is a more prominent feature of frontal lobe dysfunction and can often be one of the earliest symptoms of dementia.

ASSESSMENT

Apathy and depression can be distinguished and treated appropriately through a careful history and objective, patient-centered assessment that gathers information about previously enjoyable activities, functional performance for everyday activities, social connectedness, and the ability to work through setbacks. It is important for clinicians to work with the patient and family to create a general timeline to better understand precipitants to the loss of planning, initiating, and executing activities, with the goal of rebuilding and regaining these skills over time. Clinicians must also carefully assess for expressions of depression, sadness, shame, and self-blame with the patient and caregiver separately to account for potential difficulty in discussing these emotions.

The Apathy Evaluation Scale (AES) is an objective measurement tool to aid with evaluating for and distinguishing between apathy and depression in the elderly. The AES is a readily available, free assessment that comprises three standalone scales for the clinician (AES-C), patient (AES-S), and outside observer (AES-I), with the cumulative results considered together. It should be noted that the patient scale includes items that require insight into symptoms, and this may be impacted in cognitive disorders. A strength of the AES is its ability to differentiate probable AD dementia from clinically normal states, particularly in mild cognitive impairment (MCI) and early-stage cognitive disorders, based on the severity of apathy. With the patient, the AES-C score was 20 out of a possible 72, suggestive of very significant apathy.

To further assess depression in the geriatric population, the Geriatric Depression Scale: Short Form (GDS) is an effective and easy-to-use 15-question (yes/no response) scale to assess depression in older adults, with questions phrased in laymen's language to which older patients are able to respond more definitively than if they are asked directly if they feel depressed or sad. The GDS score in this patient was found to be 3 out of 15 (normal range), providing additional confidence that the diagnosis is apathy as opposed to depression.

Comprehensive lab results were found to be normal in this case, and these are often not helpful in differentiating apathy from depression in older patients. Further testing could include a repeat brain MRI to assess for frontal atrophy as well as further diagnostic clarification of the type of neurocognitive disorder, since in this case it appears to be a possible mixed etiology. In this case, the patient did have two positive biomarkers for ADL: hippocampal atrophy on a brain MRI and a positive amyloid positron emission tomography (PET) scan. A referral for hearing assessment resulted in a prescription for hearing aids, which helped the patient participate in conversation more readily.

TREATMENT

Apathy can be a challenge to treat, especially in more advanced stages of neurocognitive disorders when the neural circuits that drive motivation are significantly degraded. This is especially true following traumatic brain damage to frontal and subcortical connections. Getting someone involved in a structured schedule and even a day program with stimulating activities can be extremely helpful in providing external motivation. Therapeutic activities such as music, art, pet therapy, and exercise programs can be particularly stimulating to the brain. There is no specific modality of psychotherapy, however, that has specific efficacy for apathy, unless the apathy stems primarily from a mood disorder that responds to therapy.

In terms of pharmacologic management, keep in mind that stimulating medications can also overstimulate the brain, resulting in motor restlessness, agitation, and even psychosis. Sometimes the caffeine found in a morning cup of coffee or tea can be the easiest and safest way to boost someone's energy and get them engaged in activities. If a more robust pharmacologic intervention is indicated, two initial approaches are to consider either a stimulant such as low-dose methylphenidate, which has the most research supporting efficacy, or a cognitive enhancer such as memantine, which can also have stimulating effects with the additional benefit of stabilizing cognition.

Because this patient had a history of cardiac arrhythmias and low appetite, both of which could potentially be affected by a stimulant, the decision was made to first initiate memantine to target apathy. Memantine was started at 5 mg daily and titrated by 5 mg in split doses every week to a therapeutic dose of 10 mg twice daily. There was clear improvement in apathy as the patient showed an increase in initiating exercise and began walking 1 to 2 miles several times a week on her own. She was also more involved in family activities such as cooking a few dishes and helping to load and unload the dishwasher. She unfortunately experienced significant daytime fatigue on the memantine and was napping up to 2 to 3 hours daily in mid-afternoon. She was switched to the delayed-release form of memantine give at bedtime, with an observed noticeable improvement in daytime fatigue. The regular use of a continuous positive airway pressure (CPAP) machine also helped to reduce her daytime fatigue and napping.

For individuals without this patient's cardiac history, methylphenidate is a reasonable option. When methylphenidate is used, start with a low dose of 2.5 mg to 5 mg given in the morning, increasing in 5-mg increments to a total of 20 mg (in 10-mg twice-daily dosing). Methylphenidate can certainly increase blood pressure and pulse and cause overstimulation, but this is rare in the doses used for apathy. Nonetheless, it is prudent to check baseline and post-dosing vitals for a few days, and if there is a significant cardiac history to also monitor baseline and post-dosing electrocardiograms (ECGs). The stimulant Dexedrine is less commonly used but has similar effects to methylphenidate. There are numerous long-acting forms of amphetamine used to treat attention-deficit/hyperactivity disorder, but these are not recommended for use with older individuals due to the risk of side effects and persistent overstimulation.

Other potential agents that have stimulating properties in some individuals include bupropion, modafinil, and armodafinil. When used for apathy, bupropion may be dosed differently than with depression. The immediate form can be given in 37.5- to 50-mg increments by splitting a pill, and used in much the same way as methylphenidate by giving an initial morning dose and then twice daily for effect. As the dose approaches 100 to 150 mg daily using immediate-release forms and with some improvement, it may be appropriate to switch over to either the sustained-release 100-mg dose or the extended-release 150-mg formulation daily. Modafinil is dosed from 50 mg to 200 mg per day, while armodafinil is dosed from 75 mg to 150 mg daily. With any of these agents, you should be seeing some improvement in apathy within several days; if that is not the case, consider stopping them or trying something else.

KEY POINTS TO REMEMBER

- Apathy is characterized by a lack of initiation, planning, and execution of previous activities and interests, in the absence of low mood, guilt, and altered self-concept.
- The presence of depression needs to be initially assessed for and continuously monitored, as these conditions often coexist.
- A multimodal approach is often best to target apathy, including a medical work-up, pharmacologic management, use of cognitive–behavioral techniques, and working with caregivers.
- Psychotherapy can be an invaluable source of support for the patient and family, as well as collaborative care.
- Hearing and vision deficits, as well as physical weakness and all other comorbid medical concerns, should be thoroughly assessed and addressed, as they can contribute significantly to social withdrawal.

Further Reading

Budson AE, Solomon PR. *Memory Loss, Alzheimer's Disease, and Dementia: A Practical Guide for Clinicians* (2nd ed.). Elsevier; 2016.
Cipriani G, Lucetti C, Danti S, Nuti A. Apathy and dementia. Nosology, assessment and management. *J Nerv Ment Dis.* 2014;202(10):718–724.

Rosenberg PB, Lanctôt KL, Drye LT, Herrmann N, Scherer RW, Bachman DL, Mintzer JE; ADMET Investigators. Safety and efficacy of methylphenidate for apathy in Alzheimer's disease: A randomized, placebo-controlled trial. *J Clin Psychiatry*. 2013;74(8):810–816.

Ruthirakuhan MT, Herrmann N, Abraham EH, Chan S, Lanctôt KL. Pharmacological interventions for apathy in Alzheimer's disease. *Cochrane Database Syst Rev*. 2018;5(5):CD012197.

PART V

Psychotic Disorders

22 It's like she lost her mind overnight

Kripa Balaram, Deena J. Tampi, and
Rajesh R. Tampi

A 58-year-old woman is brought to the hospital
for bizarre behavior. Her family states that she
has been exhibiting irritability and mood lability
for the past week. On the day of presentation,
she began speaking of her neighbor's criminal
activity and reported having seen him talking
to his friends in his criminal ring. Her family
also report associated symptoms of increased
energy and appetite, insomnia, diarrhea, and
heat intolerance. On initial assessment, she is
tachycardic with a heart rate of 150 bpm and
hypertensive with a reading of 150/80 mmHg.
On physical examination, she has hyperreflexia
and mild diaphoresis and her thyroid gland is
nontender and enlarged.

What do you do now?

This case is an example of a patient presenting with new-onset psychotic symptoms. Psychosis is a state that can be defined as a disconnect from reality. The most common symptoms of psychosis include delusions, hallucinations, and disorganization of thought or behavior. Delusions are fixed false beliefs that can be further classified into subtypes based on their content, such as grandiose, erotomanic, persecutory, or somatic. Hallucinations are sensory perceptions that are not based in reality; they can be further classified into subtypes as well, such as auditory, visual, tactile, or olfactory. Disorganization of thought can present as bizarre behavior or speech that is incoherent or loosely associated.

Based on the presentation, you realize the importance of obtaining a thorough history. As the patient is very irritable and disorganized, she is an unreliable historian. You contact the family for further information.

Psychosis can present in the setting of a primary psychiatric illness or in the context of another medical condition. There are several theories for the etiology of psychosis occurring secondary to a medical condition. These include dopaminergic hypersensitivity, alterations in immune and oxidative processes, multifactorial genetic variability, and neurotransmitter dysfunction.

The patient's husband states that, prior to the onset of her current symptoms, she has no past psychiatric history. She has never seen a psychiatrist for any concerns and has not been admitted to an inpatient psychiatric facility. Her husband also denies any knowledge of a family history of psychiatric conditions.

When a patient presents with psychosis, there are characteristics that can suggest that the etiology is an underlying medical condition rather than a primary psychiatric diagnosis. These include no family history of psychiatric disorders, older age at onset, acute or rapid onset, the comorbid presence of medical symptoms, or the presence of atypical symptoms, such as non-auditory hallucinations.

In this case, the lack of previous psychiatric symptoms, the absence of family history, and her age all suggest that this patient has an underlying medical condition as the etiology of her current symptoms.

To identify an underlying medical condition as the cause of psychosis, a thorough diagnostic evaluation must contain all necessary components to assess for the most common etiologies. This diagnostic evaluation should include imaging, such as computed tomography (CT) or magnetic resonance imaging (MRI) of the brain, electroencephalography (EEG), and laboratory data, such as an electrolyte panel, complete blood count, liver and thyroid function tests, urinalysis or drug screen, vitamin B_{12} levels, screening for levels of common metals, HIV and syphilis, lumbar puncture, or an autoimmune panel.

CAUSES OF PSYCHOSIS SECONDARY TO A GENERAL MEDICAL CONDITION

Delirium

Delirium describes an acute confusional state that can appear most commonly in those who are hospitalized and have a history of dementia or stroke. Polypharmacy, infection, malnutrition, immobilization, or dehydration can be predisposing factors. The most common etiologies of delirium are electrolyte disturbances, substance intoxication or withdrawal, low perfusion or fluid-depleted states, infections/sepsis, hypoglycemia, or postoperative states. Patients with delirium may present with disorientation, fluctuations in awareness, distractibility, emotional lability, or agitation.

In those who are hospitalized, risk of delirium can be minimized by cognitive stimulation, maintenance of sleep/wake cycles, mobilization, and pain control. It is also important to avoid medications that can be deliriogenic, particularly in older adults. The diagnosis and management of delirium relate to identifying and treating any underlying illnesses. Acutely, the most effective interventions are often nonpharmacologic and include reorientation, mobilization, and the removal of restraints, catheters, or lines. Most individuals recover once their underlying condition has been treated and return to their previous neuropsychiatric baseline. Persistent signs of delirium have, however, been linked to poor prognosis, decreased recovery after discharge, and increased mortality.

Hepatic and Renal Disorders

Hepatic encephalopathy occurs due to liver dysfunction, such as cirrhosis. Symptoms can vary from subtle attention deficits to overt impairments in cognition, behavioral disturbances, and even coma. Hepatic encephalopathy is usually treated by alleviating underlying medical issues or inciting infections. Elevated serum ammonia levels can be treated transiently with rifaximin or lactulose. Uremia occurs due to renal dysfunction and can present with lethargy, irritability, disorientation, hallucinations, and psychosis. These signs are typically reversed by hemodialysis.

Endocrine and Metabolic Disorders

Adrenal insufficiency presents acutely with anorexia, gastrointestinal distress, confusion, or coma and can be confirmed by serum cortisol concentration and adrenocorticotropic hormone (ACTH) stimulation tests. Patients with hyperthyroidism can present with emotional lability, confusion, tremor, heat intolerance, and weight loss. Thyroid function tests and imaging can help clarify this diagnosis. The classic constellation of symptoms identifiable in primary hyperparathyroidism includes nephrolithiasis, bone resorption, gastrointestinal distress, lethargy, depression, and psychosis. Serum levels of calcium, phosphate, vitamin D, and parathyroid hormone will help to identify parathyroid disease as the underlying cause of a patient's presenting symptoms.

Porphyrias are a category of metabolic disorders characterized by dysfunction in the activities of various enzymes involved in the heme biosynthesis pathway. Although there can be variations in the presenting symptoms, porphyrias generally present with abdominal pain, peripheral neuropathy, and neuropsychiatric changes that can include confusion and psychosis. When these disorders are suspected, biochemical assays for porphobilinogens, urine/serum porphyrins, or protoporphyrin can be used. Wilson's disease, an impairment in intracellular copper transport, can present with steatosis, hepatitis, liver failure, ataxia, parkinsonism, personality changes, inappropriate behavior, and psychosis. This disorder can be diagnosed with liver function tests and copper levels.

Infectious Diseases

Various infections, such as HIV, syphilis, herpes encephalitis, and Lyme disease, can present with confusion, memory deficits, agitation, neuropathies, or psychosis. Prion disease, although rare, can also present with psychosis. A thorough work-up should include serologies and other diagnostic tests for these infectious processes. Prion diseases remain largely a diagnosis of exclusion.

Inflammatory and Autoimmune Disorders
Common types of encephalitis that can result in neurologic deficits or behavioral disturbances are usually either infectious, paraneoplastic, or autoimmune in nature. Major subtypes are listed in Table 22.1.

All these processes present with an acute to subacute onset and should be considered in any presentations of first-onset psychosis. Patients who are suspected to have either paraneoplastic or autoimmune encephalitis should have neuroimaging and EEG, but the most useful clinical tools will be lumbar puncture and cerebrospinal fluid (CSF) serology. In those with paraneoplastic encephalitis, the underlying neoplasm should also be identified and addressed. In general, a treatment approach consists of immunosuppressive therapy with glucocorticoids, intravenous immunoglobulin, plasmapheresis, or cytotoxic therapy. Other autoimmune conditions, such as lupus, multiple sclerosis, and chronic meningitis, can also present with behavioral changes and neuropsychiatric symptoms.

Neurodegenerative Disorders
Although the predominant deficits seen in neurocognitive disorders are memory and complex cognitive function, there can often be psychiatric changes. All the most common types of neurocognitive

TABLE 22.1 **Encephalitides associated with psychosis**

Paraneoplastic encephalitides	Autoimmune encephalitides
Anti-Hu receptor (SCLC)	Anti-NMDA, anti-LGI1, anti-Caspr2, anti-AMPA receptor, anti-GABA A receptor, anti-GABA B receptor, anti-IgLON5, anti-DPPX, anti-GlyR, anti-mGluR1 and anti-mGluR5, anti-neurexin-3 alpha, anti-GFAP antibody
Ma2-associated (testicular cancer)	
Anti-CRMP (SCLC or thymoma)	
Other types: limbic, brainstem, encephalomyelitis, myelitis	

disorders—Alzheimer's dementia, vascular dementia, Lewy body dementia, Parkinson's disease, progressive supranuclear palsy, normal pressure hydrocephalus, and Creutzfeldt–Jakob disease—have some form of behavioral disturbance. Assessment should include physical examination, extensive neurologic/neuropsychological testing, and neuroimaging. Antipsychotic medications can be used for behavioral disturbances, but they should be used cautiously and preferably for as short a time as possible. Other effective nonpharmacologic interventions include maximizing family involvement and providing psychosocial support.

Other Neurologic Processes

Patients who present acutely after a traumatic brain injury (TBI) or cerebrovascular accident can exhibit episodes of confusion, disorientation, agitation, or aggression. Agitation and aggression are most common in the "awakening" phase immediately after a TBI; appropriate options for treating acute agitation include rapid-onset antipsychotic medications, mood stabilizers, benzodiazepines, and agents like amantadine, buspirone, and beta-blockers. New-onset psychiatric symptoms can also be seen with space-occupying lesions, any process causing brain tissue herniation, brain or neuroendocrine tumors, or central nervous system cysts.

Vitamin Deficiencies

Vitamin B_{12} and folic acid deficiencies are commonly associated with neuropathy and gait disturbances, depression, insomnia, cognitive slowing, and even frank psychosis. Thiamine deficiency, commonly seen in those with alcohol use disorder, can also present with psychiatric symptoms. Korsakoff syndrome, which arises in the setting of persistent thiamine deficiency, can present with amnesia, confabulation, and confusion. Unlike with vitamin B_{12} or folic acid deficiency, repletion usually will not completely resolve the symptoms of thiamine deficiency, and most patients require some form of rehabilitation.

Medications or Other Substances

The most common medications that can cause behavioral changes are anabolic steroids, corticosteroids, analgesics, anticholinergic and antiparkinsonian agents, antivirals, and immunotherapy. Some medications can negatively affect older adults in greater proportion. Intoxication or withdrawal from various substances can also cause psychiatric symptoms.

Based on her examination and vitals, this patient may have thyroid dysfunction. Complete metabolic panels, thyroid function tests, toxicology screen, and an electrocardiogram (EKG) are obtained. Her EKG shows tachycardia with a regular rhythm and her thyroid function demonstrates elevated T_3/T_4 and decreased thyroid-stimulating hormone (TSH) levels. These values indicate a state of hyperthyroidism. Given her current symptoms, you arrive at a diagnosis of thyroid storm.

As with all other psychiatric conditions, the clinician's priority is to minimize the risk of harm to the patient or others. When psychosis secondary to a medical condition is suspected, treating the underlying condition will generally result in resolution of symptoms. Neuropsychiatric symptoms that exist transiently or emergently should be treated with antipsychotics or benzodiazepines. A specific treatment regimen that aligns with an individual patient's needs, comorbidities, and preferred administration modality can be used. If mood symptoms are also present, treatment with antidepressants or mood stabilizers can be initiated. Families must be educated on the underlying medical disorder, accompanying psychiatric disturbances, and effective nonpharmacologic management.

Patients presenting with psychosis may also require acute inpatient psychiatric hospitalization for crisis stabilization or to prevent the risk of harm to self or others while a diagnostic work-up is completed and a treatment regimen is finalized.

After discussing this diagnosis with the patient and her family, you initiate a treatment regimen for hyperthyroidism and refer the patient to endocrinology for further management. For transient treatment of her psychosis and for acute symptoms of agitation, you prescribe haloperidol 5 mg orally twice daily. You explain to the patient and her family that antipsychotics are a short-term addition to the treatment plan until her thyroid function is regulated.

KEY POINTS TO REMEMBER

· Neuropsychiatric symptoms can develop due to a primary psychiatric condition or in the setting of another medical condition,

- When a patient presents with new-onset psychosis, it is essential to perform a thorough history and physical examination and a detailed diagnostic work-up.
- Treatment of the underlying medical condition usually resolves any psychiatric symptoms that are present.
- Transiently, any acute symptoms can be managed with antipsychotics or benzodiazepines.
- Patients may also require inpatient psychiatric hospitalization for acute stabilization and to minimize the risk of harm to self or others.

Further Reading

Colijn MA, Nitta BH, Grossberg GT. Psychosis in later life. *Harvard Rev Psychiatry.* 2015;23(5):354–367.

Cummings J, Pinto LC, Cruz M, Fischer CE, Gerritsen DL, Grossberg GT, Hwang T-J, Ismail Z, Jeste DV, Koopmans R, Lanctot KL, Mateos R, Peschin S, Sampaio C, Tsuang D, Wang H, Zhong K, Bain LJ, Sano M. Criteria for psychosis in major and mild neurocognitive disorders: International Psychogeriatric Association (IPA) consensus clinical and research definition. *Am J Geriatr Psychiatry.* 2020;28(12):1256–1269.

Keshavan MS, Kaneko Y. Secondary psychoses: An update. *World Psychiatry.* 2013;12(1):4–15.

23 She thinks I'm someone else

Silpa Balachandran, Deena J. Tampi, and Rajesh R. Tampi

A 78-year-old woman is brought to the emergency department (ED) after complaints from the neighbors about loud noises coming from her home. The emergency response team found the woman to be very agitated and verbally aggressive and accusing her husband of attempting to poison her. At the ED, her vital signs were in the normal range. Physical and neurologic examinations are unremarkable.

You find the woman sitting calmly in her bed. She greets you pleasantly and agrees to talk to you about this ED visit. During your conversation, her mood changes abruptly and she accuses you of wanting to kill her. She gets increasingly agitated, but she settles down when directed. She tells you that for some time another person who resembles her husband has been living in her house and is always watching her. This is why she lashed out at her husband and also feels that her neighbors are involved.

What do you do now?

This case is a description of an older adult presenting with psychotic symptoms. "Psychosis" is not defined as a disease entity in the major psychiatric classification systems but rather as representing specific symptoms within other disorders, including delusions (false, fixed beliefs, often of a bizarre nature), hallucinations (false sensory perceptions, commonly either visual or auditory in older adults), disorganized thinking, and grossly disorganized motor behavior (including catatonia), or negative symptoms such as blunting of affect and poverty of speech and thought. Regardless of the etiology, psychotic features among older adults are often difficult to differentiate and treat, resulting in frequent hospitalizations, institutionalization, and increased caregiver burden and burnout. They also increase the risk of morbidity and mortality for the older adult. Understanding the etiology for the psychotic symptoms is crucial in deciding on the treatment plan for these symptoms.

The initial question would be whether the symptoms of psychosis are due to a primary psychotic disorder such as schizophrenia or if they are secondary to a medical or neurologic disorder, including delirium, Parkinson's disease, dementia, stroke, adverse medication effects, or the effects of substances of abuse. A detailed history can help us make this distinction.

Based on your understanding of a need for a more detailed history, you get in touch with the patient's husband.

The acuity of the onset of psychotic symptoms is generally an excellent indicator of etiology. Acute or subacute onset of symptoms might suggest a secondary cause for the psychosis (e.g., delirium with an onset of days to weeks or medication/substance-induced psychosis with an onset of days to months). Neurocognitive disorders (NCDs), on the other hand, may present with psychotic symptoms that tend to have an insidious onset of symptoms that may take months to years to manifest. Do not always presume that reports of persecution are delusional in nature; make sure to rule out elder abuse if there telltale signs of abuse or neglect.

You are not able to reach the husband immediately, so while waiting to hear back you order some tests to rule out secondary causes of psychosis.

Complete blood count (CBC), complete metabolic panel (CMP), thyroid-stimulating hormone (TSH), vitamin B_{12}, folate level, syphilis antibodies, erythrocyte sedimentation rate (ESR), urine toxicology, autoimmune panels, and HIV tests are ordered and eventually come back as non-revelatory. You review her medication list and find nothing of significance. You decide to hold off on computed tomography (CT) and magnetic resonance imaging (MRI) of the head as it is a low-yield investigation given the absence of focal neurologic findings.

The patient's husband informs you she was diagnosed with Alzheimer's dementia 7 years earlier. Her dementia symptoms have been worsening over the last few years. He confirms that the patient has never been diagnosed with any other psychiatric conditions in the past. You realize the patient is describing persecutory delusions, visual hallucinations, and misidentification in the setting of a major neurocognitive disorder (very likely Alzheimer's disease [AD]), which has progressed in severity over the past 7 years. You also consider other differential diagnoses as NCD can be due to multiple etiologies. The most common ones are Alzheimer's dementia, vascular dementia, frontotemporal dementia (FTD), dementia associated with Lewy body disease, and Parkinson's disease. Other differentials to consider are neurodegenerative diseases and reversible causes of dementia.

PSYCHOSIS IN AD

Psychosis in AD is now considered a primary manifestation of underlying pathology. Suggested diagnostic criteria for psychosis in AD include the presence of hallucinations and delusions in a patient who has previously met all requirements for AD; symptoms that are severe enough to disrupt the function of the patient or others and are present for ≥1 month, at least intermittently; and symptoms that are not attributable to delirium, other medical conditions, drug effects, schizophrenia, or other primary psychiatric disorders.

Psychotic symptoms are quite common in AD, with a prevalence estimated at slightly higher than 40%. The risk of psychosis is higher with greater degrees of cognitive decline, and in individuals of African American or Black ethnicity. Persecutory delusions and visual hallucinations are common psychotic symptoms, while auditory hallucinations tend to be rare. Psychosis is also associated with a faster rate of cognitive decline among individuals with AD.

PSYCHOSIS IN OTHER NCDS

Psychotic symptoms are seen in approximately 15% of individuals with vascular dementia and present similarly as in AD. In dementia with Lewy bodies, the prevalence of psychosis is much higher, with rates of hallucinations at 78% and delusions at 25%. Auditory hallucinations are less common than visual hallucinations and delusions. In FTD, delusions do occur, but less frequently than in AD, and hallucinations are much less common. The prevalence of psychosis in FTD is approximately 10%, with higher prevalence among individuals with genetic mutations of chromosome 9 open reading frame 72 (C9ORF72) and granulin (GRN). Delusions, hallucinatory behavior, and suspiciousness are present in one-fifth of patients with the behavioral variant of FTD, whereas negative psychotic symptoms such as social and emotional withdrawal, blunted affect, and formal thought disorders are more frequently (≥80%) seen among these individuals.

Approximately 20% to 60% of Parkinson's disease patients may report psychotic symptoms, of which the most common are visual hallucinations and delusions. The psychotic symptoms are often caused by side effects of various antiparkinsonian medications, including levodopa, dopamine receptor agonists, the dopamine-releasing drug amantadine, and the monoamine oxidase inhibitor selegiline. Thus, reviewing the patient's medication list is of high importance.

The timing of the onset of psychotic symptoms is variable in different major NCDs. Among individuals with AD, psychotic symptoms often appear much later during the course of the illness, unlike in individuals who have Lewy body dementia, in which well-formed visual hallucinations are found to occur early on. Table 23.1 provides an overview of the presentation of psychosis across the major forms of NCDs.

You have now ruled out other secondary causes of psychosis and are considering different approaches to managing her psychotic symptoms.

TABLE 23.1 **Psychosis in major subtypes of NCDs**

Type of NCD	Alzheimer's dementia	Vascular dementia	Dementia with Lewy bodies	FTD
Features	Poor short-term memory; slow progressive decline	Underlying history of atherosclerotic disease; poor learning curve; psychomotor slowing; relative preservation of language skills. Stepwise progressive decline.	Impaired visuospatial and executive function, fluctuating attention, concentration; visual hallucinations; Parkinsonian motor symptoms; frequent falls	Early loss of personal and social awareness; hyperorality; stereotyped, perseverative behavior
Frequency of psychosis	Common	Common	Common	Less common
Type and onset of psychosis	Visual hallucinations and delusions occur later.	Visual hallucinations and delusions occur later.	Well-formed visual hallucinations occur early on with the onset of illness.	Paranoia, auditory hallucinations (more common in C9ORF72 mutation carriers) and negative symptoms of psychosis (affective flattening, alogia, avolition) may be present for only a short period to re-emerge later or occur later during disease course.

TREATMENT

Nonpharmacologic interventions remain the mainstay of treatment for non-urgent neuropsychiatric symptoms, and guidelines suggest limiting pharmacologic interventions to severe, dangerous, or highly distressing symptoms. The most consistently effective interventions have focused on home-based caregivers and aim to develop their skills, improve their general well-being, and reduce their perceived burden. These caregiver-related outcomes are predictive of whether a patient with dementia can remain in the community or will be transitioned to institutional care.

No medications have approval from the U.S. Food and Drug Administration (FDA) for the treatment of the psychotic symptoms of NCDs. When medication is required, clinicians are encouraged to follow the "3T" approach: (1) *target* specific symptoms, (2) *titrate* dosage based upon clinical response and tolerability, and (3) *time-limit* medication use to avoid unnecessary treatment. Regardless of the underlying disease, there are no perfect options when it comes to pharmacotherapy. The choice of treatment often comes down to finding a medication that maximizes symptomatic improvement while minimizing adverse effects. The second-generation antipsychotics risperidone (0.25–1 mg), olanzapine (2.5–10 mg), quetiapine (25–200 mg), aripiprazole (2–10 mg), and brexpiprazole (2–4 mg) have all shown some evidence of efficacy for the treatment of agitation and psychosis in AD and vascular dementia. However, the effects are variable and the treatment of psychotic symptoms (vs. agitation alone) might require aiming for the higher end of the listed dosing ranges.

In patients with Lewy body dementia, cholinesterase inhibitors are initially favored over antipsychotics as psychotic symptoms appear to result from cholinergic neurodegeneration and not hyperdopaminergic activity. In this case, donepezil (5–10 mg), rivastigmine (6–12 mg), and galantamine (8–16 mg) are all viable agents, and should be titrated into therapeutic ranges. When there is a lack of effect, second-generation antipsychotics can be considered. On the one hand, there is a paucity of data concerning the safety and efficacy of antipsychotics among these individuals and a clearly elevated risk of severe side effects, including parkinsonism, sedation, and even delirium. Nonetheless, clinicians often turn to antipsychotics to treat persistent and disruptive symptoms such as delusions of misidentification, which can lead to severe agitation and resistance. Low-dose quetiapine

(25–100 mg) is often used given its lower potency and weaker D2 receptor binding compared to risperidone, despite the fact that other studies indicate that antipsychotic effects in AD may require dosing in the 200-mg range. Risperidone has much tighter D2 receptor binding and should be used with great caution and in the lowest dosing ranges (0.25–0.5 mg). Better options may include olanzapine (up to 5 mg) or even clozapine (12.5–50 mg). Clozapine has greater serotonergic affinity and selective binding of D1 mesolimbic receptors while sparing striatal D2 receptors. The challenge with the use of clozapine is its significant adverse-effect profile, including sedation, orthostatic hypotension, and agranulocytosis, which limits its use.

Currently there are no FDA-approved pharmacologic therapies for FTD. In FTD patients with severe behavioral disturbances who may require an antipsychotic medication, second-generation antipsychotics with fewer extrapyramidal side effects are preferred. Agitation may be controlled by atypical antipsychotics such as risperidone, olanzapine, quetiapine, and clozapine, but the clinician should carefully monitor for adverse effects. Antipsychotics have been suggested to be more helpful in treating psychotic symptoms in patients with the C9ORF72 subtype of FTD.

The cardiovascular, cerebrovascular, metabolic, and extrapyramidal adverse effects of antipsychotics are particularly concerning when these medications are used among older adults. Additionally, the small (2.0–3.7%) but significant increase in the absolute risk of all-cause mortality associated with their use can be worrisome for patients and caregivers. The FDA boxed warning indicating an association between the administration of antipsychotics in geriatric patients and increased mortality risk must be kept in mind when prescribing antipsychotics to older adults for any reason. Given these concerns, a risk/benefit conversation for using antipsychotics should be completed and documented with patients and their caregivers. Additionally, the lowest effective doses of medications should be used to control the psychotic symptoms. The clinical utility of using the antipsychotics should be re-evaluated every 3 to 4 months or sooner as indicated. If the individual does not respond to the medication or develops adverse effects, it should be stopped.

Based on your understanding of these issues, you have a long discussion with the patient's husband and children. They understand the risks and benefits and choose a pharmacologic approach to treat her hallucinations. You recommend low-dose risperidone starting at 0.5 mg orally daily. She tolerates risperidone well and is discharged back to her home with recommendations to follow up with you in 2 to 4 weeks.

KEY POINTS TO REMEMBER

- Psychotic symptoms are a part of the natural course of most major NCDs.
- History is helpful in distinguishing different types of major NCDs that cause psychotic symptoms.
- Nonpharmacologic treatment is first-line management strategy.
- There are no FDA-approved medications to treat psychotic symptoms in NCDs.
- Second-generation antipsychotics can be used with caution to treat psychotic symptoms in NCDs due to AD, vascular dementia, and behavioral variants of FTD.
- Antipsychotics are best avoided in psychosis due to Lewy body dementia.

Further Reading

Gossink FT, Vijverberg EG, Krudop W, Krudop W, Scheltens P, Stek ML, Pijnenburg YA, Dols A. Psychosis in behavioral variant frontotemporal dementia. *Neuropsychiatr Dis Treat.* 2017;13:1099–1106.

Nagahama Y, Okina T, Suzuki N, Matsuda M, Fukao K, Murai T. Classification of psychotic symptoms in dementia with Lewy bodies. *Am J Geriatr Psychiatry.* 2007;15:961–967.

Reus VI, Fochtmann LJ, Eyler AE, Hilty DM, Horvitz-Lennon M, Jibson MD, Lopez OL, Mahoney J, Pasic J, Tan ZS, Wills CD, Rhoads R, Yager J. The American Psychiatric Association practice guideline on the use of antipsychotics to treat agitation or psychosis in patients with dementia. *Am J Psychiatry.* 2016;173:543–546.

Ropacki SA, Jeste DV. Epidemiology of and risk factors for psychosis of Alzheimer's disease: A review of 55 studies published from 1990 to 2003. *Am J Psychiatry.* 2005;162: 2022–2030.

Stinton C, McKeith I, Taylor JP, Lafortune L, Mioshi E, Mak E, Cambridge V, Mason J, Thomas A, O'Brien JT. Pharmacological management of Lewy body dementia: A systematic review and meta-analysis. *Am J Psychiatry.* 2015;172:731–742.

He is frightened of things that he sees

Arshiya Syeda Farheen, Deena J. Tampi, and Rajesh R. Tampi

A 69-year-old man with past history of Parkinson's disease (PD) for 14 years is brought to the emergency department (ED) by his family members for worsening symptoms of visual hallucinations over the past year. He sees children in his backyard, and he believes that they want to hurt him. In the ED he is found to be agitated and frustrated that his family members don't believe what he is seeing. He is currently being treated with levodopa/entacapone/carbidopa and ropinirole for the management of PD. The patient is admitted to the medical floor for further work-up. You are consulted to manage his agitation and address his visual hallucinations. The patient appears anxious and paranoid. ." On the cognitive examination, he is alert and oriented to time, place, and person. On examination, his vital signs are in the normal range and he has cogwheeling rigidity in both arms and he walks with a shuffling gait.

What do you do now?

This case is a typical presentation of PD psychosis (PDP) based on demographics, medical history, medications, and physical examination, including the cogwheeling rigidity, shuffling gait, unilateral pill-rolling tremor, and gradual onset of visual hallucinations. The prevalence of psychosis in cross-sectional studies of individuals with PD is 13% to 60% depending on the selected diagnostic criteria and the specific population. The lifetime prevalence of psychosis in PD is 47% to 60%. The symptoms of psychosis vary across the course of PD. Early symptoms experienced include passage hallucinations (where a person, animal, or indefinite object is seen briefly passing in the peripheral visual field), illusions (for example, seeing the branch of a tree as a cat), and presence hallucinations (a feeling that someone is nearby). Pareidolia refers to a specific class of illusion where faces and objects are seen in formless visual stimuli, such as clouds, flames, or tree bark, or in geometric visual patterns, such as carpets or wallpaper. This can occur as a normal perceptual experience but is increased in frequency in PD and related disorders such as dementia with Lewy bodies. The prevalence of minor phenomena among individuals with PD is 20% to 45%, co-occurring with hallucinations in 13% to 27%.

Visual hallucinations are the most common feature of PDP, in contrast to primary psychotic disorders, where auditory hallucinations are most common. Hallucinations are more frequent in dim lighting or at the end of the day. The patient's retention of insight into these hallucinations may fluctuate over time and may be related to the degree of concomitant cognitive impairment. Delusions are less frequent than hallucinations in PDP. When present, delusions are most commonly paranoid in nature, and the most common theme is infidelity.

Dopamine has been most consistently recognized as an important neurotransmitter for development of psychosis. The most commonly explained mechanism of PDP is centered on the dopaminergic medications used for the motor symptoms of PD, which increases the sensitivity of dopamine in the mesolimbic and mesocortical areas, especially the ventral striatum. The mechanism by which anti-parkinsonism drugs increase the patient's susceptibility to psychosis involves hypersensitization of dopamine receptors in the nigrostriatal pathway, leading to dysfunction of limbic structures. All medications used to treat PD, including dopaminergic medications, levodopa, and non-dopaminergic medications such as anticholinergics, amantadine, and monoamine oxidase B inhibitors, are associated with the development of PDP. However, dopamine alone does not always appear to be the initiating factor. The loss of serotonergic neurons in the raphe nucleus may lead to hypersensitive serotonin receptors in the prefrontal cortex; this in turn leads to glutamate hyperactivity and resultant activation of the mesolimbic pathways—implicated in PDP as described earlier.

ASSESSMENT

After a thorough history from the patient and a focused physical examination, the next step is gathering collateral information from the family. The patient's family informs you that the patient started having visual hallucinations at night 1 year ago. They have gradually progressed to occurring both at night and during the day. Their intensity has also increased, and now the patient is paranoid that the unknown kids are conspiring to kill him.

At this point, it is imperative to perform a more detailed mental status examination to test for attention, concentration, and memory. Relevant lab studies should be obtained, including a complete blood count, electrolytes, renal and liver function tests, calcium, thyroid-stimulating hormone, vitamin B_{12} and folate levels, and a urinalysis. More detailed lab studies should be based on the clinical presentation and history. Neuroimaging would be indicated if the clinical examination reveals focal neurologic findings. These lab studies and other relevant tests may indicate other causes for the psychosis, such as delirium related to a variety of metabolic, toxic, or infectious causes, or acute drug intoxication (e.g., alcohol, cocaine, amphetamine, hallucinogens). The psychosis could also be due to other forms of dementia, including progressive supranuclear palsy, corticobasal degeneration, or dementia with Lewy bodies. Psychotic symptoms due to primary or comorbid psychiatric conditions must be reviewed. For example, late-onset bipolar disorder and major depressive disorder with psychotic symptoms are usually distinguished by mood-congruent symptoms (e.g., delusions of guilt, worthlessness in the case of psychotic depression) in the context of prominent affective symptoms. In contrast, patients with PDP typically have psychotic symptoms unrelated to mood (e.g., seeing cats running on the bed). Other differential diagnoses include brief psychotic disorder, delusional disorder, and substance-induced psychosis.

TABLE 24.1   **NINDS–NIMH diagnostic criteria for PDP**

Symptoms that are recurrent or persistent for >1 month	Symptoms include illusions, presence hallucinations, hallucinations (visual, auditory, olfactory), delusions
Type and onset of psychosis	Gradual; begins with presence hallucinations to progress to visual hallucinations and delusions
Exclusion of other probable diagnoses	· Dementia with Lewy bodies · Late-onset psychosis · Delirium · Organic brain lesions · Other neurocognitive disorders

In this case, the psychotic symptoms were clearly associated with the progression of PD and did not appear to have other explanations.

In 2007 a work group from the National Institute of Neurological Disorders and Stroke (NINDS) and the National Institute of Mental Health (NIMH) proposed new diagnostic criteria for PDP. The diagnosis requires the presence of characteristic psychotic symptoms that develop following the onset of PD, persist either continuously or recurrently for at least 1 month, and are not more likely to be secondary to an alternative diagnosis. These criteria are detailed in Table 24.1.

MANAGEMENT

It is crucial to treat the psychotic symptoms promptly and completely since they can otherwise reduce the patient's quality of life and increase the patient's level of disability; can increase the safety risk for the patient and caregivers; and can increase caregiver burden. Consult the neurologist managing the neurologic symptoms of PD to review the patient's PD medications, and consider trying to minimize or reduce the dose of agents that may be causing psychosis. This must be carefully done as the same medications that control symptoms of PD can trigger psychotic symptoms.

Antipsychotic medications are often used as first-line treatments for PDP, even though they have limited efficacy and carry a high risk for side effects, such as worsening motor symptoms. Quetiapine is often used as a first-choice drug since it is the least potent in terms of D2 receptor binding and may pose the lowest risk of extrapyramidal symptoms; at the same time, it can be sedating and at higher does it can pose an increased risk for falls. Risperidone, olanzapine, and aripiprazole are also common choices but are accompanied by a higher risk of extrapyramidal symptoms. In two randomized controlled trials, clozapine was found to be effective for the treatment of PDP without worsening motor function. However, its use is limited due to agranulocytosis. In a randomized open-label trial of 45 patients with PDP, clozapine and quetiapine were shown to be equally effective in reducing psychotic symptoms, as measured by the Brief Psychiatric Rating Scale (BPRS), but several subsequent randomized controlled trials demonstrated no change in psychotic outcomes with quetiapine. Despite the lack of convincing evidence for the efficacy of quetiapine, it is preferred over clozapine in low doses for treating PDP given the risk of agranulocytosis and need for extensive monitoring for clozapine.

Pimavanserin is the first atypical antipsychotic medication that has approval from the U.S. Food and Drug Administration (FDA) for the treatment of hallucinations and delusions associated with PDP. It exhibits selective 5-HT2A inverse agonist activity with much lower affinity for 5-HT2C receptors and negligible D2 and histamine receptor activity. It has been proved to be safe, effective, and well tolerated, with high antipsychotic activity, and lacks the side effects, such as sedation or motor impairment, usually seen with other available antipsychotics.

Because of the close association between severe hallucinations in PD and dementia, cholinesterase inhibitors may be effective in the context of preexisting visual hallucinations or PD with dementia. A 24-week study of rivastigmine for PD dementia among outpatients found improvement in visual hallucination incidence.

Electroconvulsive therapy (ECT) has shown to be effective not only for the treatment of PDP but also for the motor symptoms of PD. However, ECT should only be considered when pharmacologic treatments have failed, if there are intolerable side effects, or if there are clear contraindications.

After a risk/benefit analysis and discussion with the patient, his family. and his neurologist, you decide to start this gentleman on a low dose of quetiapine. His agitation, visual hallucinations, and paranoia improve within 2 days after starting the quetiapine. The patient is discharged home with outpatient neurology and psychiatry follow-up.

KEY POINTS TO REMEMBER

- PDP is a common condition and is associated with increased morbidity, mortality, and caregiver burden among individuals with PD.
- Rule out other medical causes and medication effects for psychosis before making the diagnosis of PDP.
- Decreasing the number and dosage of anti-PD drugs could alleviate the PDP symptoms but may worsen motor function.
- Clozapine is proven to be effective in PDP, with fewer side effects than quetiapine. However, the use of clozapine is limited due to potentially lethal agranulocytosis and the need for extensive monitoring.
- Pimavanserin, a serotonin receptor inverse agonist, is FDA approved in the United States to treat PDP.

Further Reading

Fénelon G, Mahieux F, Huon R, Ziégler M. Hallucinations in Parkinson's disease: Prevalence, phenomenology and risk factors. *Brain.* 2000;123(4):733–745.

Fénelon G, Soulas T, Zenasn F, De Langavant LC. The changing face of Parkinson's disease-associated psychosis: A cross-sectional study based on the new NINDS-NIMH criteria. *Mov Disord.* 2010;25(6):763–766.

Gama RL, de Bruin VM, de Bruin PF, Távora DG, Lopes EM, Jorge IF, Bittencourt LR, Tufik S. Risk factors for visual hallucinations in patients with Parkinson's disease. *Neurol Res.* 2015;37(2):112–116.

Lee AH, Weintraub D. Psychosis in Parkinson's disease without dementia: Common and comorbid with other non-motor symptoms. *Mov Disord.* 2012;27(7):858–863.

Sahli ZT, Tarazi FI. Pimavanserin: Novel pharmacotherapy for Parkinson's disease psychosis. *Exp Opin Drug Discov.* 2018;13(1):103–110.

Schneider RB, Iourinets J Richard IH. Parkinson's disease psychosis: Presentation, diagnosis and management. *Neurodegen Dis Manag.* 2017;7(6):365–376.

25 Suspicious neighbors

Michael Reinhardt, Muniza A. Majoka, and Marco Christian Michael

A 67-year-old woman was brought into a clinic by her husband, who had become increasingly concerned about her behavior, stating, "We need help . . . this is not how my wife is." Five months ago, the woman retired from a long career in law enforcement. Since then she had begun to experience progressive anxiety regarding her neighbors, eventually developing a belief that they had been surveilling her. The neighbors in question lived directly across the street from her and had vehemently denied all surveillance. The woman had repeatedly confronted them regarding her beliefs and constructed her own countersurveillance apparatus. The persistence of her actions had led the neighbors to threaten legal action. The woman's husband has described her as having difficulties with attention, handling her daily affairs, and depression that have all worsened, along with her paranoid thoughts.

What do you do now?

This case paints an intriguing clinical scenario of an aging patient presenting with new-onset psychotic symptoms, depression, and possible cognitive impairment in late life. Specifically, the patient appears to have developed a delusion (fixed false belief) that her neighbors are surveilling her. In search of clarity, the clinical team must work to establish a firm diagnosis through careful clinical assessment. Accurate diagnosis greatly impacts outcome in cases like this, as treatment varies tremendously across the potential differential diagnoses.

Approximately 60% of psychotic states presenting in late life are attributable to secondary causes (e.g., major neurocognitive disorder, delirium, substance use, medication adverse events, and other medical/neurologic conditions) rather than primary mental illness (e.g., schizophrenia, schizoaffective disorder, delusional disorder, major depressive disorder, bipolar disorder). To clarify the underlying condition with the patient, then, the initial evaluation should include thorough patient and collateral histories, physical and neurologic examinations, laboratory testing, and a cognitive assessment.

HISTORY, PAST AND PRESENT

On further exploration of her history, this was the woman's first psychiatric consultation. She reported no prior psychopharmacologic treatment. The patient and her husband both endorsed a long history of increased vigilance, particularly regarding perceived threats to the safety of their family. This vigilance became more pronounced after joining the police department. The patient had always regarded this as a "healthy paranoia," which had never impaired her work or home life. Over the past 5 months, however, the patient had become increasingly preoccupied by her persecutory delusion, at times ignoring her obligations while obsessing over the neighbor's surveillance. She denied auditory or visual hallucinations but did state "I see the glint of the binoculars in their window!" repeatedly during the assessment. The patient and husband denied symptoms of mania, panic attacks, generalized worry or tension, and obsessive thoughts or compulsions, but did endorse changes to her "focus" and some difficulty handling daily affairs. Furthermore, over the past month she had also begun to complain of worsening depression, stating, "I am just trying to keep them safe; why don't they believe me?" However, she denied suicidal ideation or plan. The family noted that she did have access to a firearm (a handgun) for which she was fully licensed.

Her past medical history included only hypertension, controlled via lifestyle interventions and diet. She had no history of seizure disorder, traumatic head injury, neurotoxic exposures, autoimmune conditions, or endocrine disorders. Her medication profile included a daily multivitamin and low-dose aspirin. She drank alcohol socially very intermittently and denied any history of cigarette or illicit drug use. Regarding her social history, she was a college-educated woman, with no adverse childhood events or developmental delays. There were vague reports of paranoia in her father but no confirmed family history of mental illness; there was a maternal history of Alzheimer's disease (AD) with onset at age 93.

EXAMINATION

On mental status examination, the patient was fully oriented to time, place, and self. She was a pleasant and neatly groomed woman dressed in a gray pants suit. She was cooperative with the interview and was without psychomotor abnormalities. She maintained eye contact and her speech was unremarkable. Her mood was "stressed"; her affect was mildly dysphoric, constricted but reactive and appropriate. Her thought process was linear and goal directed. Her thought content was significant for the persecutory delusion, but she denied other delusions (control, somatic, grandiose, nihilistic, misidentifications) and denied thought broadcasting or insertion. She denied suicidal or homicidal ideation or plans. She denied visual, auditory, tactile, and gustatory hallucinations. She had limited insight and limited judgment regarding her delusion but intact judgment in other areas of function.

Her physical examination was remarkable only for being slightly overweight, while her neurologic examination was wholly unremarkable with normal cranial nerve function, no focal weakness, no tremor, and no gait abnormalities. During her initial appointment, she was administered a comprehensive cognitive battery to assess her complaints of forgetfulness and inattention. The cognitive battery revealed mild impairments in attention and working memory, with normal performance in all other domains of cognition, including short-term memory, visuospatial function, abstraction, praxis, and executive function. She *scored an 8 on the Hamilton Depression Rating Scale, indicating mild depression. Laboratory testing was noncontributory, revealing normal blood counts, thyroid function, electrolytes, liver function, vitamin B_{12} and D levels, metabolic function, and infectious disease screening. Magnetic resonance imaging of the brain without contrast revealed periventricular white matter changes and age-related volume changes without significant atrophy.*

Given our available data, the patient's condition is not explained by her known medical conditions or pharmacotherapy, diminishing the likelihood of a psychotic disorder due to another medical condition or a substance- or medication-induced psychotic disorder. This would increase the diagnostic probability of a primary psychotic disorder—particularly delusional disorder, given her non-bizarre delusion. The patient's complaints of inattention and forgetfulness in combination with the family history of AD in a first-degree relative raises the specter of a mild or major neurocognitive disorder (3% to 14% prevalence of psychosis in minor neurocognitive disorder and 10% to 73% prevalence of delusions in AD). The presence of depression (15% to 45% prevalence of psychosis in late-life depression) and premorbid paranoid personality traits further complicate the diagnostic picture.

Following this comprehensive assessment, all secondary psychotic disorders were ruled out. The patient did not meet full criteria for schizophrenia or schizoaffective disorder given the lack of hallucinations, bizarre delusions, disorganization of speech or behavior, and negative symptoms. She did not meet full criteria for a personality disorder, but did meet criteria for both delusional disorder and major depressive disorder. Furthermore, the chronology of this case indicated a newly incident delusion that was followed approximately 4 months later by depression without a history of mania or hypomania, excluding both major depressive disorder with psychotic features and bipolar disorder as primary diagnoses.

DEFINING THE DIAGNOSIS

Delusional disorder across the lifespan is often accompanied by deficits in attention and working memory, as was the case for this patient. Delusional disorder is a rare condition, with an estimated prevalence of 0.03% among older adults. It generally has an onset in midlife to late life, presents with an isolated delusion, and is associated with social dysfunction, cognitive complaints, and difficulties in personal and occupational functioning. Risk factors include a paranoid personality, genetic vulnerabilities, adverse childhood events, and socioeconomic factors. Major depressive disorder is comorbid with delusional disorder in up to a third of cases and contributes to an elevated risk of suicide. Unfortunately, individuals with delusional disorder have, by definition, minimal to no insight into the delusional nature of their thinking, which severely limits engagement with treatment. As the patient stated: "I am not sick. I am just trying to keep my family safe. Why don't they believe me?"

MANAGEMENT

The patient's symptoms were causing significant disruptions to her social functioning and had begun to have legal ramifications. Given the severity of her illness, antipsychotic treatment was warranted, but it was rejected by the patient, who didn't believe she had a psychiatric illness. After extensive psychoeducation and repeated demands by her family and legal team, the patient acquiesced to attending psychotherapy. She was referred for Cognitive Behavior Therapy for Psychosis (CBT-P) with the targeted hope of developing insight into her condition.

There are limited data to support the efficacy of psychotherapy in the treatment of delusional disorder in any age group; however, cognitive–behavioral therapy and its variants are perhaps the best-studied form of therapy for this population. CBT-P is focused on the resolution of psychotic symptoms by engaging the patient in a three-step process targeted at developing insight and alternative explanatory models for delusional beliefs. A similar therapeutic model, Cognitive Behavior Social Skills Therapy (CBSST), which merges cognitive–behavioral therapy with social skills training, has shown benefit in schizophrenia in late life and might also have been considered in this case.

The patient attended CBT-P for 6 consecutive weeks and had modest improvement in her symptoms before suffering a setback when she received an adverse ruling in the legal case brought against her by her neighbors. Over the next 4 weeks, she began to complain of worsening depression and was re-evaluated. She was again screened with the Hamilton Depression Rating Scale and her score had risen to a 36, indicating severe depression. She had become hopeless regarding her situation and had begun to contemplate suicide, planning to end her life with her handgun. Her persecutory delusion also returned to its original severity; she believed that her suspicions were confirmed by the lawsuit's outcome. Her condition necessitated emergent psychiatric hospitalization. During her psychiatric admission, the patient begrudgingly agreed to start taking an atypical antipsychotic medication in combination with an antidepressant. Upon careful consideration, risperidone and escitalopram were chosen as her medications.

There are limited data to guide the choice of treatment in delusional disorder in older adults. The available studies suggest that outcomes, including sustained remission, are improved with the use of an atypical antipsychotic. Choice of an atypical antipsychotic is guided by expert consensus, with preference (in descending order) for risperidone (0.75 to 2.5 mg daily), olanzapine (5 to 10 mg daily), and quetiapine (50 to 200 mg daily). A treatment choice must then be made according to each patient's unique presentation and comorbidities. Medication dosing must be minimized in late-life psychotic disorders to limit extrapyramidal, metabolic, and other side effects.

The patient was started on risperidone 0.25 mg daily, which was titrated to 0.5 mg after 7 days. Escitalopram 5 mg daily was initiated and titrated to 10 mg after 1 week. She was discharged from the hospital after a 14-day stay, markedly improved and without further suicidal ideation or plan. The patient and her family agreed to turn in her handgun to the local police department out of an abundance of caution. After discharge, the patient continued her medications and resumed CBT-P with her therapist. She continued to gradually improve over the next 6 months. The deficits in attention and working memory noted on initial evaluation improved modestly on retesting but did not objectively or subjectively resolve.

As is common with delusional disorder, the patient had two further recurrences of her illness over the next several years, necessitating brief increases in risperidone dosage and booster sessions of CBT-P. In general, recurrence rates may be limited but not entirely obviated by treatment. She also suffered from further recurrences of major depressive disorder surrounding each episode. At the age of 75, she began to suffer from increasing deficits in short-term memory and was eventually diagnosed with AD. This development is consistent with a potentially increased risk of AD in patients with delusional disorder, necessitating regular assessment of cognitive status.

- Delusional disorder in older adults is a diagnosis of exclusion, necessitating comprehensive evaluation before diagnosis with this primary psychiatric illness.
- Delusional disorder in older adults may be accompanied by cognitive deficits in working memory and attention that warrant further surveillance, as these patients may be at increased risk for progressive cognitive decline.
- Patients with delusional disorder suffer from increased rates of major depression, placing them at increased risk for suicide.
- While data are limited, the best available evidence suggests that patients benefit from combined treatment strategies that include an atypical antipsychotic (risperidone, olanzapine, or quetiapine) and therapy (CBT-P or CBSST).

Further Reading

Copeland JR, Dewey ME, Scott A, Gilmore C, Larkin BA, Cleave N, McCracken CF, McKibbin PE. Schizophrenia and delusional disorder in older age: Community prevalence, incidence, comorbidity, and outcome. *Schizophr Bull*. 1998;24(1):153–161.

Granholm E, McQuaid JR, McClure FS, Auslander LA, Perivoliotis D, Pedrelli P, Patterson T, Jeste DV. A randomized, controlled trial of cognitive behavioral social skills training for middle-aged and older outpatients with chronic schizophrenia. *Am J Psychiatry*. 2005;162(3):520–529.

Jalali Roudsari M, Chun J, Manschreck TC. Current treatments for delusional disorder. *Curr Treat Options Psych*. 2015;2(2):151–167.

O'Connor K, Stip E, Pelissier MC, Aardema F, Guay S, Gaudette G, Van Haaster I, Robillard S, Grenier S, Careau Y, Doucet, P, Leblanc V. Treating delusional disorder: A comparison of cognitive-behavioural therapy and attention placebo control. *Can J Psychiatry*. 2007;52(3):182–190.

Reinhardt MM, Cohen CI. Late-life psychosis: Diagnosis and treatment. *Curr Psychiatry Rep*. 2015;17(2):1.

Tampi RR, Young J, Hoq R, Resnick K, Tampi DJ. Psychotic disorders in late life: A narrative review. *Ther Adv Psychopharmacol*. 2019;9:2045125319882798.

26 I live with these voices

Tarek K. Rajji

A 75-year-old woman has a 45-year history of schizophrenia. She is single, has never been married, and is supported by her brother and government resources. She lives in a group home and follows up regularly at an outpatient geriatric psychiatric clinic for the past two decades. While she is relatively independent with her basic daily functioning, she needs assistance for more complex tasks such as managing her personal affairs and finances. After several failed antipsychotic trials in her 40s, she has been maintained since her 50s on olanzapine 20 mg daily. Still, she continues to experience auditory hallucinations of family members from childhood talking to her at times, but these voices are not distressing or command in nature. Over several weeks, the patient's counselor and group home administrator noticed that she has been more forgetful and at times confused. They also noted worsening of her psychotic symptoms and more behavioral response to internal stimuli.

What do you do now?

Individuals with schizophrenia aged 55 years or older will soon account for 25% or more of the total schizophrenia population. The prevalence of schizophrenia in older adults is expected to double and reach 1.1 million people in the United States by 2025 and 10 million worldwide by 2050. Notwithstanding the personal and family burden of schizophrenia among older adults with schizophrenia, the economic costs of the illness are as high in late life as in a first episode.

Most older adults with schizophrenia have had their illness since early adulthood, although a minority have a late onset (defined as ages 40 to 60; about 24%) or a very late onset (older than 60; about 3%). In longitudinal studies, between 46% and 84% of patients with schizophrenia have been reported to experience significant clinical improvement, and 21% to 77% some social recovery. However, about 20% remain institutionalized or quasi-institutionalized, with the rest living mainly in the community.

There are several key differences between early- and late-onset schizophrenia. Later-onset schizophrenia is seen more in women and is characterized by more positive symptoms (e.g., delusions, hallucinations, thought disorder) than negative symptoms (e.g., apathy, withdrawal, affective blunting). Emergent cognitive deficits associated with late-onset schizophrenia show more variability across cognitive domains, versus more generalized deficits seen among those with an earlier onset. Finally, patients with late-onset schizophrenia tend to respond to lower doses of medications than those with an early onset.

SYMPTOMS AND TREATMENT WITH AGE

A common belief is that as individuals with schizophrenia age, positive symptoms become milder and negative symptoms and cognitive impairment emerge and dominate the clinical presentation. Recent evidence suggests, however, that there is quite a bit of fluctuation in all of these symptoms through the late decades of life. Still, for patients with persistent or emerging positive symptoms, antipsychotic medications continue to be the mainstay of treatment. However, it is critical to remember that older adults with schizophrenia are likely to require much lower doses of antipsychotic medications and that they are more susceptible than younger individuals to adverse effects. The different response of older adults with schizophrenia to antipsychotic medications is due to age-related pharma-cokinetic changes, such as a higher volume of distribution and elimination half-life and an increase in blood–brain barrier permeability. It is also due to pharmacodynamic changes resulting from lower availability and sensitivity of dopaminergic D2 receptors in the brain. In one study, older adults with schizophrenia who were stable on a fixed dose of olanzapine or risperidone had their dose reduced by 40% with excellent tolerability and reduction in extrapyramidal side effects.

Higher doses of antipsychotic medications in older individuals can have disproportionately adverse effects on negative symptoms and cognitive changes, due to excessive dopamine receptor blockade as well as anticho-linergic and antihistaminic effects. Clozapine and olanzapine, in particular, have a high anticholinergic burden. Thus, it is recommended to use lower doses in older adults with schizophrenia, and start with medications that have less anticholinergic burden, such as aripiprazole, risperidone, or ziprasidone. In addition, keep in mind that aging individuals with schizophrenia can also develop dementia, putting them at greater risk of antipsychotic-associated cerebrovascular accidents, pneumonia, and even mortality.

With age, negative symptoms may have more clinical impact than pos-itive symptoms. These symptoms may not change over time, and there are no consistently effective treatments for them. However, being aware of these symptoms and appreciating the fact that some of them may be secondary to the antipsychotic medications patients are using is another reason why reducing the dose of antipsychotic medications may be indicated clinically in stable patients with persistent negative symptoms.

COGNITIVE DEFICITS

Cognitive deficits in schizophrenia are core features of the illness, are observed across the lifespan, and are among the strongest predictors of functional decline in this population. Older adults with schizophrenia have significant cognitive deficits in almost all cognitive domains, including attention/vigilance, executive function, learning and memory, speed of processing, and working memory. Functional impairment and decline is closely associated with these deficits. There seems to be heterogeneity in the trajectory of cognitive function in older adults with schizophrenia based on residential status. The rate of cognitive decline in community-dwelling older adults with schizophrenia appears to be similar to the rate of cognitive decline among older healthy adults despite the fact that they are impaired at any time point. In contrast, chronically institutionalized older adults with schizophrenia experience an acceleration of cognitive decline around age 65. This difference could be due to difference in cognitive reserve between the two populations. Finally, some studies suggest also a fluctuating course over time late in life. In addition, older adults with schizophrenia have a two-fold increased risk of developing frank neurocognitive disorders such as vascular dementia or Alzheimer's disease before the age of 80 years when compared with the general population. One large cohort study that reviewed a Medicare database over 10 years found that at age 66 nearly 30% of individuals with schizophrenia had a comorbid diagnosis of dementia compared to less than 2% of those with a serious mental illness. A comparable rate of dementia is not seen in persons without schizophrenia until they are in their late 80s.

To date there are no effective treatments for cognitive deficits in older adults with schizophrenia. Cognitive remediation and training programs that have shown some benefit among younger adults appear to be less effective in the older population. Cognitive enhancers used in dementia such as acetylcholine esterase inhibitors have also not been shown as effective. Thus, it remains critical to focus on reducing iatrogenic burden on cognition, especially from medications with high anticholinergic, antihistaminic, and anti-dopaminergic burden, as they all have been associated with impaired cognition in these individuals. Among those with schizophrenia and comorbid dementia, psychosocial interventions that focus on cognitive, behavioral, functional, and social skills training as well as on management of chronic health comorbidities have shown promise to enhance function and overall quality of life.

MORBIDITY AND MORTALITY

While the number of older adults with schizophrenia is growing along with the growth of the general aging population, their life expectancy continues to be shorter compared to their peers by about 15 years. This gap has been increasing over the past decades as individuals with schizophrenia do not seem to be benefiting from the advances in medicine that are contributing to longer life expectancy in the general population. Some of the main reasons for death in these aging individuals with schizophrenia include suicide, accidents, congestive heart failure, and chronic obstructive pulmonary disease. Their medications and lifestyle, including poor diet, high rates of smoking, and physical inactivity, also contribute significantly to their shorter life expectancy. Other key factors include poor access to general medical care due to stigma and lack of adequate collaborative care among mental health and medical professionals.

Thus, it is important to conceptualize schizophrenia in late life as a chronic medical condition in which optimal management includes an integration of physical and mental health treatments as well as adequate access to both and psychosocial rehabilitation.

Due to her increased psychotic symptoms, the patient's psychiatrist initially increased her antipsychotic medication olanzapine, only to find her doing worse and becoming more confused. On the one hand, her increased forgetfulness and general cognitive decline was not new, and appeared to be related to both her increased negative symptoms (apathy and social withdrawal) and her increasing age. A neuropsychological assessment showed poor effort and interest in the testing as well as deficits across several domains. At the same time, these and other psychotic symptoms appeared to worsen acutely several weeks after the patient abruptly stopped smoking due to a worsening chronic cough and shortness of breath. Both her psychiatrist and her primary care doctor wondered if she was more confused due to an increase in the blood levels of olanzapine following smoking cessation. The olanzapine dose was reduced gradually to 10 mg per day, and her confusion as well as her positive psychotic symptoms improved, although she still had noticeable negative symptoms and cognitive impairment. It was decided to begin regular skills training with a counselor and in groups to improve her social and functional abilities.

KEY POINTS TO REMEMBER

· Schizophrenia persists into late life but can also start in later life. Later-life onset is more common in women and is associated with positive symptoms such as delusions and hallucinations.

- Negative symptoms tend to be more common in late life and include apathy, social withdrawal, and affective blunting.
- Although mild forms of cognitive impairment can be seen across the age spectrum in schizophrenia, they are more common and impactful in late life and come with an increased risk of neurocognitive disorders.
- Schizophrenia in late life is comparable to many chronic medical conditions, and optimal management requires adequate access to integrated medical and psychiatric services.

Further Reading

Cohen CI, Vahia I, Reyes P, Diwan S, Bankole AO, Palekar N, Kehn M, Ramirez P. Focus on geriatric psychiatry: Schizophrenia in later life: Clinical symptoms and social well-being. *Psychiatr Serv.* 2008;59:232–234.

Graff-Guerrero A, Rajji TK, Mulsant BH, Nakajima S, Caravaggio F, Suzuki T, Uchida H, Gerretsen P, Mar W, Pollock BG, Mamo DC. Evaluation of antipsychotic dose reduction in late-life schizophrenia: A prospective dopamine D2/3 receptor occupancy study. *JAMA Psychiatry.* 2015;72:927–934.

Putnam KM, Harvey PD. Cognitive impairment and enduring negative symptoms: A comparative study of geriatric and nongeriatric schizophrenia patients. *Schizophr Bull.* 2000;26:867–878.

Rajji TK, Mulsant BH. Nature and course of cognitive function in late-life schizophrenia: A systematic review. *Schizophr Res.* 2008;102:122–140.

Rajji TK, Mulsant BH, Nakajima S, Caravaggio F, Suzuki T, Uchida H, Gerretsen P, Mar W, Pollock BG, Mamo DC, Graff-Guerrero A. Cognition and dopamine D2 receptor availability in the striatum in older patients with schizophrenia. *Am J Geriatr Psychiatry.* 2017;25:1–10.

White KE, Cummings JL. Schizophrenia and Alzheimer's disease: Clinical and pathophysiologic analogies. *Compr Psychiatry.* 1996;37:188–195.

PART VI

Other Disorders

27 Suddenly not the same

Ipsit V. Vahia

A 72-year-old woman with major neurocognitive disorder is brought in for a psychiatry assessment because her daughter has noticed that her behavior "seems to have changed over the past week or so." She reports that the patient's confusion has worsened and that though she appears alert, she does not directly respond to questions until and that she has been answering in monosyllables. On one evening, she suddenly became agitated and yelled at a peer for no discernible reason. According to her daughter, these behaviors are unusual for her. The daughter also reports that she spoke to her mother but says that the conversation was quite coherent.

What do you do now?

ASSESSING AND DIAGNOSING DELIRIUM

Delirium is a commonly seen and frequently underdiagnosed clinical syndrome in older adults. It is characterized by an acute decline in cognition and attention. Its clinical presenting features include a combination of fluctuating levels of alertness and consciousness and acute onset of cognitive decline, including deficits in orientation, memory, attention, and language. It is also characterized by alterations in behavior that may include worsening agitation, aggression, hallucinations (most commonly visual), and paranoid ideation. However, in many cases behavioral symptoms may also include apathy, psychomotor retardation, and amotivation; this syndrome is frequently referred to as "hypoactive delirium." The delirium syndrome can also include disruptions in sleep and lability of mood.

There is no definitive diagnostic test for delirium, and identifying it depends on astute clinical observation along with a detailed clinical history that includes information from the past days to weeks. Because of the fluctuating patterns of clinical symptoms, it is not unusual for patients to present with intermittent periods of lucidity. Episodes of agitation or apathy and confusion may be interspersed with periods of calm and controlled behavior and clear, if transient, insight. In assessing suspected delirium, it is important to obtain as much collateral information as possible from reliable informants or caregivers. A detailed physical and neurologic examination is also essential, since it can help distinguish delirium from common confounding conditions such as dementia, depression, or psychosis. It may also help detect signs of conditions such as trauma.

Over the past decade, there has been increased use of specially developed and well-validated screening instruments such as the Confusion Assessment Method (CAM), which can indicate the potential presence of delirium and trigger appropriate investigation and examination.

Delirium is typically observed secondary to an organic trigger. While its mechanisms are not fully understood, it is now widely accepted as resulting from the interaction of multiple factors. These include preexisting risk factors such as dementia, frailty, and multiple medical comorbidities. It is usually triggered by precipitating factors such as a new acute medical condition (e.g., an infection) or a new medication that may cause a drug interaction leading to delirium. Thus, assessment of a patient presenting with suspected delirium involves a thorough physical examination as well as lab tests to identify potential causes. Vital signs including core temperature and blood oxygenation levels may provide valuable information on underlying general medical conditions. While the lab tests ordered should be determined by the history and physical examination, a standard panel may include a complete blood count (CBC), a metabolic panel that includes hepatic and renal function tests, levels of thyroid-stimulating hormone (TSH), vitamin B_{12} and folic acid levels, and a urinalysis and culture. In specific circumstances, tests such as the erythrocyte sedimentation rate (ESR) or C-reactive protein levels may be appropriate. A chest X-ray may be ordered if a pulmonary infection is suspected. An electrocardiogram (EKG) may shed light on cardiopulmonary causes. Neuroimaging may be considered if the neurologic examination indicates focal neurologic deficits.

Aside from the major neurocognitive disorder, the patient has no other relevant neuropsychiatric history. She is also in relatively good physical condition; her only comorbidity is hypercholesterolemia, which is well controlled on 20 mg rosuvastatin. Aside from this and supplements of vitamin B_{12} and folic acid, she is taking no additional medications.

Upon interview, the patient appears somewhat lethargic and is not very engaged in conversation, but she does smile and respond when asked a direct question, albeit in one- or two-word answers. Her daughter says that her mother is usually quite verbal and this represents a notable change from her baseline. Her physical exam is unremarkable, but an attempt to perform a cognitive screening task is not successful because the patient declines to perform tasks or ask questions, simply shaking her head.

EPIDEMIOLOGY AND PREVENTION

Because delirium is a frequent occurrence among older adults, it should be suspected whenever a change in behavior is noted among older adults, especially those with concurrent medical conditions. The incidence of delirium among medical inpatients can be as high as 30%. Among those in intensive care units (ICUs), the prevalence can be as high as 80%. Among older adults in non-hospital settings, community prevalence rates may be as high as 15% among those in their 80s. For those in hospice care, the prevalence may be as high as 30%. Delirium must also be considered when assessing patients living at long-term care facilities or nursing homes, where its prevalence is estimated to be between 30% and 60%.

Prevention remains the cornerstone of management of delirium. In managing older adults, an assessment of risk factors is important. This begins with determining functional status and functional independence. Older adults with limited ambulation, advanced dementia, and inability to manage activities of daily living (ADLs), as well as those demonstrating frailty or malnutrition, may be more likely to develop delirium in the face of medical or physiologic triggers. For older adults in high-risk environments such as hospitals, nursing homes, or residential facilities, a combination of nonpharmacologic interventions targeting risk factors for delirium may be effective in prevention. This may include management of pain, measures to minimize infection risk, ensuring adequate nutrition and hydration, assistance with ambulation, and monitoring sleep as applicable.

Careful review of both psychotropic and non-psychotropic medications and preempting potential drug interactions is also essential. A careful review of all medications is a core component of evaluation of a person with acute confusion. Of particular relevance is the need to identify whether any medications may have an anticholinergic effect, since anticholinergic medications are among the most common precipitants of delirium. Clinicians should aim to minimize the overall psychotropic medication load. This may involve discontinuing nonessential medications or reducing the doses so that any essential psychotropic medications are administered at the lowest possible dose. There is a very broad list of medications that can trigger delirium within specific contexts. For instance, diuretics administered to manage conditions like congestive heart failure may trigger delirium by leading to dehydration. There are, however, certain classes of medications that are particularly well-documented triggers for delirium. Sedative medications (e.g., benzodiazepines), opioid analgesics, and anticholinergic medications used to manage allergies (e.g. diphenhydramine) are the most frequent causes of delirium.

As such, any medication with the ability to cross the blood–brain barrier has the potential to trigger or worsen delirium. This includes not only all psychiatric medications but also medications used for neurologic conditions (e.g., antiparkinsonian drugs, anticonvulsants, medications for migraine). Evaluation of delirium should also include an assessment of over-the-counter drugs. Several liquid formulations that include alcohol may cause delirium, and many formulations of medications for common conditions such as cough or congestion have anticholinergic properties. In addition to this, consideration must also be given to a person's use of alcohol, tobacco, and cannabis products or other controlled substances, all of which may trigger or worsen delirium.

Finally, polypharmacy is an independent risk factor for delirium. From the perspective of identifying triggers, managing ongoing delirium, and reducing the risk of future episodes of delirium, attention must be paid to whether a given patient's medication load can be reduced. This may be accomplished by identifying and changing medications that may impact each other, eliminating ineffective or suboptimally dosed medications, and reducing dosages where possible so that medications are used at the minimum necessary dose.

MANAGEMENT

While the management of delirium may vary depending on the clinical setting in which it is detected, certain common principles apply.

Identify and Treat the Underlying Etiology
As mentioned earlier, the cornerstone of managing delirium is to identify and treat the underlying cause. This may involve a range of approaches depending on the cause. Infections should be treated with appropriate antibiotics. If pain is a factor, adequate pain management should be implemented. Adequate nutrition and hydration is also important.

Appropriate Supportive Care
Supportive steps to prevent delirium in high-risk patients are also a key to management. This involves maintaining a consistent routine, ensuring adequate sleep and nutrition, repeated orientation by staff, one-on-one care to the extent possible, and maintaining ambulation and self-care.

Pharmacologic Management
In general, the use of psychotropic medications should be minimized, as noted earlier. However, in patients with acute behavioral agitation,

resistance to care, psychosis, or disorganization, it may be necessary to use psychotropic medications. Antipsychotics are the most frequently used agents, with haloperidol use supported by the largest body of literature. While older adults are at a higher risk of extrapyramidal side effects, the use of antipsychotics to manage delirium is usually short term. Starting at a small oral dose (as low as haloperidol 0.5 to 1 mg) and slowly increasing the dose until the adequate therapeutic effect is achieved may be an appropriate strategy. Other antipsychotics such as risperidone or olanzapine may also be effective. When patients exhibit a severe enough delirium that oral administration of medications may not be feasible, intramuscular antipsychotics may be considered. In persons exhibiting severe agitation within ICU or inpatient hospital settings, intravenous antipsychotic use may also be considered.

Monitoring Response

Management of delirium involves close monitoring of patients. Because delirium is typically a syndrome with medical and psychiatric aspects, it is best managed by interdisciplinary teams that can simultaneously assess and treat underlying medical conditions, manage behavioral symptoms, and provide the appropriate level of supportive care. As such, plans for delirium management should be tailored to each individual, depending on their general condition, cognitive status, and ability to actively participate in their own care. Typically, daily monitoring of vital signs, repeating lab tests as indicated, and monitoring medication combinations are all part of the process of monitoring ongoing response to care. Of note, it is common for symptoms of delirium to resolve several days or even weeks after the underlying medical cause is identified and successfully treated. In some cases, the symptoms of delirium (especially hypoactive delirium) may persist for weeks and even a few months after the patient is successfully treated.

SPECIAL CONSIDERATIONS

Prognosis

The long-term outcomes of delirium may vary considerably based on a person's general medical condition and functional status. Overall, however, delirium is associated with increased mortality. Hyperactive delirium is associated with worse outcomes than hyperactive delirium. Prolonged delirium and situations where delirium symptoms do not fully resolve are also associated with worse outcomes. In persons who are in hospice care, the onset of delirium without a clearly identified trigger is often an indication of approaching end of life.

Relationship with Dementia

It has been suggested that persons experiencing delirium may be at higher risk of developing dementia in the longer term. However, this relationship has not been definitively demonstrated. It is also unclear what the causal direction is. While some believe that delirium causes disruptions of neural architecture that may trigger dementia, others have suggested that delirium is more frequent in persons with underlying dementia pathology, even prior to onset of any cognitive symptoms.

Relationship with COVID-19

During the global COVID-19 pandemic, delirium was frequently the primary presenting symptom among older adults infected by the SARS CoV-2 virus. It is common for delirium to be the only presenting symptom among older adults with COVID-19, and it can predate the emergence of respiratory and flu-like symptoms by several days. As a result, COVID-19 is considered part of the standard protocol of investigation for any older adult with acute confusional symptoms. Keep in mind, however, that it is not uncommon for older adults with COVID-19 to test negative during initial presentation despite the presence of delirium. In instances where COVID-19 infection is an active risk, standard precautions must be taken by any provider caring for an older adult with delirium symptoms.

Although a physical examination and blood tests are unremarkable, urinalysis indicates the presence of a urinary tract infection. While you await the results of urine culture and sensitivity testing, her primary care provider prescribes an antibiotic. After 48 hours, results of culture indicate that her infection is sensitive to the antibiotic. You follow her longitudinally and note that over the next 4 weeks, her symptoms resolve and she returns to her baseline.

- Delirium is a common condition in older adults, especially those with multiple medical comorbidities, and manifests as an acute confusional state with accompanying behavioral symptoms.
- Delirium is especially common among older adults with medical comorbidities and requires a thorough clinical assessment with collateral history from reliable informants, detailed physical examination, monitoring vital signs, and lab assessments to identify underlying organic etiology.
- The occurrence of delirium is much higher among older adults who are hospitalized, who are living in nursing homes or long-term care facilities, and who are taking multiple medications.
- Management of delirium depends primarily on nonpharmacologic approaches including supportive care, eliminating triggers, and careful management of sleep, nutrition, and hydration.
- Psychotropic medications may be considered for acute agitated behavioral symptoms, but their use should generally be minimized.

Further Reading

Alagiakrishnan K, Wiens C. An approach to drug-induced delirium in the elderly. *Postgrad Med J*. 2004;80:388–393.

Kalish VB, Gillham JE, Unwin BK. Delirium in older persons: Evaluation and management. *Am Fam Physician*. 2014;90(3):150–158. [Erratum in *Am Fam Physician*. 2014;90(12):819.]

Oh ES, Fong TG, Hshieh TT, Inouye SK. Delirium in older persons: Advances in diagnosis and treatment. *JAMA*. 2017;318(12):1161–1174.

It's just a nightcap

Luminita Luca and Elizabeth A. Crocco

An 83-year-old man presents to the clinic with insomnia and poor concentration. He expresses dissatisfaction with his life because he feels slowed down by age. He is asking for meaning in his life. He admits having one or two glasses of whiskey before going to bed to help him relax. In the past year, he has increased his drinking to three glasses of whiskey nightly. He does not believe anything is wrong with this increased consumption of alcohol, and says he came to the appointment mostly to appease his wife. He admits to some forgetfulness, which he thinks is part of growing old. He is in good health, apart from a heart condition and peripheral neuropathy. He was recently prescribed low-dose gabapentin for his neuropathy and zolpidem for insomnia. He has slight tremors in both hands, which he says are inherited from his father.

What do you do now?

Alcohol use represents a significant problem in older adults. According to the 2013 National Survey on Drug Use and Health, more than half of elderly subjects report having used alcohol in the past month; more than 4% endorsed heavy use. One drink, or 0.5 oz of alcohol, constitutes approximately 1.5 oz of liquor, 12 oz of beer, or 5 oz of wine. For men and women above 65 years of age, one daily drink is considered moderate drinking, more than two drinks daily represents heavy drinking, and four or more drinks in one sitting is considered bingeing. The patient meets criteria for heavy drinking for someone his age. This may be surprising for him as well as for his healthcare providers, who may view one glass of red wine a day as beneficial. Overall, drinking patterns established earlier in life tend to persist in older men but less so in women. Notable risk factors for alcohol abuse in older adults include a family history of alcoholism, previous episodes of alcohol or drug use, insomnia, depression, and chronic pain. As in this patient, alcohol is used to self-medicate insomnia and anxiety and may be masking clinical depression.

Benzodiazepines are commonly prescribed by physicians, although only one-third of these prescriptions might be appropriate. With long-term benzodiazepine use, characterized as continued daily use for longer than 3 months, problems are more likely to arise, including dependence, increased risk for falls, and cognitive deficits. Illicit substance use in older adults is higher in the United States compared to other countries, yet clinicians may easily overlook it. Results from the 2012 National Survey on Drug Use and Health revealed that 7.2% of individuals above age 50 used illicit substances, an increase from previous years. This effect is driven by the baby boomers, individuals born during the post-World War II years, who have now become senior citizens. Similar to their younger counterparts, cannabis is the most commonly used illicit drug among older adults. Its medical use has become accepted with the relaxation of legislative restrictions. Older adults who use cannabis are more likely to be men, living alone, and with depressive symptoms. Opiate use is mostly due to prescription abuse rather than illicit drugs. Cocaine and stimulants are used by 0.7% of senior adults; they are more likely to be men with multiple medical comorbidities.

KEY CONCEPTS IN SUBSTANCE USE

Clinicians commonly use descriptors such as "abuse," "dependence," and "substance use disorder" to describe clinically relevant alcohol and drug addiction. The International Statistical Classification of Disease and Related Health Problems (ICD-10) includes diagnoses of harmful use or abuse (a pattern of recurrent use leading to distress and interpersonal consequences) and dependence (when patients develop tolerance, withdrawal, or inability to control the intake). The distinction between abuse and dependence was eliminated in the most recent edition of the American Psychiatric Association's *Diagnostic and Statistical Manual of Mental Disorders* (DSM-5) and was replaced with the broader terminology of substance use disorder (SUD). SUD describes a wide range of clinically relevant symptoms, with severity ranging from mild to severe. The term "addiction," not included in either the DSM-5 or ICD-10, is used by clinicians to describe severe presentations. Other descriptors such as "at risk" and "heavy" drinking indicate a likelihood to develop unintended consequences or physical dependence.

This patient has tremors and the inability to cut down on his alcohol use, which are both signs demonstrating a high likelihood that he meets criteria for an alcohol use disorder. As a result, further questioning and evaluation is warranted.

MEDICAL CONSEQUENCES

With age, metabolism slows down and the ability to clear alcohol is reduced. Acute alcohol consumption impairs liver function, and chronic use can induce malnutrition through impaired absorption, vitamin deficiencies, and low albumin. In any work-up for SUD, serum levels of thiamine, folate, and B_{12} need to be evaluated. Alcohol can reduce adherence to medication regimens during binge-drinking episodes. Benzodiazepines, particularly those with long half-lives, deposit in fat tissue, which increases significantly with aging in relation to lean body mass. This accumulation of drug increases the risk for sedation as well as respiratory depression, particularly in patients with chronic pulmonary conditions.

Elderly individuals can be predisposed to falls due to decreased muscle strength or arthritis. Alcohol adds to the risk for falls through its diuretic effect, resulting in low blood pressure and dizziness. Chronic alcoholics develop ataxia with wide-based gait due to peripheral sensory neuropathy and cerebellar atrophy. Benzodiazepines produce a similar effect of unstable gait and sedation.

The patient has an unspecified neuropathy, which is possibly a consequence of alcohol use. He is drinking a heavy amount of alcohol and routinely taking zolpidem, a non-benzodiazepine hypnotic, which has an additive effect on sedation and increased risk for falls.

The aging alcoholic patient carries risk factors for brain injury and dementia. Having a significant history of alcohol use in middle age increases the risk of dementia two-fold. Comorbid smoking, hypertension, vitamin deficiencies, and head trauma all contribute to the risk of brain injury and resultant cognitive impairment seen in elderly drinkers. Additionally, Wernicke–Korsakoff syndrome is seen with heavy alcohol use. In the acute phase, Wernicke encephalopathy is characterized by altered mental status, ataxia, and oculomotor disturbances. If left untreated, patients progress to Korsakoff syndrome, with anterograde and retrograde amnesia and executive dysfunction, which are chronic and irreversible. The cognitive deficits seen in Wernicke–Korsakoff syndrome are a direct consequence of acute thiamine deficiency, which is commonly seen in heavy alcohol users with poor nutrition, although alcohol's direct neurotoxic effects also add to the risk of cognitive impairment.

The patient's long history of alcohol use and falls should alert the clinician to evaluate both cognitive status and potential cognitive risk factors that can be modified.

DIAGNOSIS

Clinicians often do not suspect alcohol or drug abuse as a significant contributor to dysfunction in older adults and are more likely to suspect medical illnesses alone. Additionally, patients are often reluctant to disclose patterns of abuse, or may minimize their habits. Due to co-occurring medical problems, elderly patients are more likely to suffer from protracted symptoms of withdrawal or failure to respond to detoxification treatment.

TABLE 28.1 **Symptoms of substance abuse in older patients**

Physical symptoms	Cognitive problems
· Ataxia, impaired gait, frequent falls	· Sedation
· Slurred speech	· Disorientation
· Bruises	· Forgetfulness, memory deficits
· Tremors	
· Tachycardia, high blood pressure	
· Seizures	
· Cardiomyopathy	
· Liver disease, cirrhosis	
· Gastrointestinal disease	
· Cancer	
· Weight loss, deconditioning	
Psychiatric symptoms	**Social problems**
· Excessive anxiety	· Job loss
· Insomnia	· Social isolation
· Depressed mood	· Financial losses
· Irritability	· Interpersonal problems with families
· Perceptual disturbances	· Institutionalization

Additively, use of alcohol or other substances makes recovery from medical illness more difficult. Common symptoms associated with alcohol and drug abuse in older adults are listed in Table 28.1.

Screening for alcohol and substance use should be part of any routine clinical evaluation in the geriatric population. The CAGE-AID questionnaire is a brief, easy-to-administer screening instrument for alcohol and drug use that is useful in a busy clinical setting. Blood tests can offer strong evidence of recent use (e.g., blood alcohol level [BAL]) or chronic use (e.g., increased levels of gamma glutamyl transferase [GGTP] and carbohydrate deficient transferrin [CDT]). Urine tests are useful in screening and monitoring for concurrent drug use.

The patient had a CAGE score of 2, suggestive of high-risk drinking. He would benefit from further clinical evaluation.

Identifying abuse of benzodiazepines and non-benzodiazepine sedative–hypnotics is challenging, as these drugs are often prescribed by a practitioner. Benzodiazepine toxicity is characterized by sedation, ataxia, and slurred speech. Chronic users of benzodiazepines and non-benzodiazepine sedative–hypnotics can present with frequent falls, ataxia, cognitive deficits, sedation, and disinhibition. Urine toxicology confirms the presence of benzodiazepines. The patient's chronic use of zolpidem, in addition to alcohol, places him at higher risk for significant adverse effects.

Despite recent relaxed legislation, cannabis poses significant risks for older adults. It is known to increase respiratory rate, induce tachycardia, elevate blood pressure, and increase the risk of acute heart events. Cannabis can induce cognitive blunting as a long-term effect in older adults.

As seen in younger patients, opiates intended as short-term interventions for pain may lead to chronic use in older adults as well. Opiate dependence in older adults is manifested by anxiety, tachycardia, and diarrhea, symptoms that are nonspecific and may be attributable to a variety of medical conditions. Overt withdrawal can develop within hours of opioid cessation and presents with runny nose, restlessness, and abdominal pain. A thorough review of the current medications is essential to identify opiates that may be leading to these symptoms. Dependence and withdrawal are best avoided when the prescribing physician institutes short-term treatment with opiates and has a clear discontinuation plan.

TREATMENT

Patient with SUDs require a thorough evaluation by a clinician with correct identification of the co-occurring psychiatric conditions, such as depressive disorders, anxiety, and sleep problems. Substance abuse often represents an attempt to self-medicate for depression or dysphoria. Because the patient reports having anxiety, he may benefit from treatment of any underlying anxiety disorder with an antidepressant (e.g., a serotonin specific reuptake inhibitor [SSRI] or serotonin–norepinephrine reuptake inhibitor [SNRI]), rather than a benzodiazepine anxiolytic. Zolpidem should be slowly tapered and removed. Deprescribing benzodiazepines and opiates is the ultimate goal in any SUD treatment.

Most patients with substance abuse complain of insomnia, which may persist long after abstinence has been achieved. Pharmacologic options to target insomnia include melatonin, ramelteon (a melatonin receptor agonist), and small doses of sedating antidepressants such as mirtazapine and trazodone. Hypnotics and anticholinergics (e.g., diphenhydramine, hydroxyzine) should be avoided due to side effects such as dizziness, falls, and worsening cognition.

Acute Treatment of Withdrawal

Alcohol withdrawal must be identified and treated promptly. Typical symptoms include confusion, disorientation, anxiety, tremors, autonomic instability, and elevated blood pressure. Tachycardia, which is typically found in young patients, may not be present in older individuals due to atrioventricular block and antihypertensive use. Delirium with overt visual hallucinations occurs in about 5% of patients with alcohol use disorder, yet in older adults a more common situation is protracted withdrawal, with subtle signs of anxiety and mild tremors, or a more prolonged recovery from a medical condition for which the patient is receiving treatment.

Alcohol withdrawal is best treated in a specialized inpatient service for select elderly patients. Treatment should include supportive oral or parenteral hydration, correction of electrolyte abnormalities, vitamin supplementation, and short-term use of a benzodiazepine. Due to age-related slowing of hepatic metabolism, shorter-acting benzodiazepines (e.g., lorazepam, oxazepam) are favored over longer-acting ones (e.g., chlordiazepoxide, diazepam), which accumulate in the fatty tissue with resulting excessive sedation. For mild forms of dependency, outpatient treatment with supervised pharmacotherapy can be successful.

Benzodiazepine withdrawal, sometimes complicated with delirium or seizures, may occur when benzodiazepines are abruptly discontinued. Benzodiazepine cessation protocols are used in hospital settings to control acute withdrawal symptoms. The treatment of uncomplicated benzodiazepine dependence consists of slow, controlled reduction of the daily dose over time, sometimes months, to avoid discomfort.

Overt opiate withdrawal is best treated in a medical setting due to risks for dehydration. A recent Canadian guideline recommended buprenorphine–naloxone as the first-line option for opioid withdrawal management in older adults.

Maintenance Treatment

Patients completing alcohol and drug detoxification programs require further treatment and a multifaceted approach, including pharmacotherapy, psychotherapy, community-based interventions, and family support. These interventions are targeted toward reducing relapse. Naltrexone (an opiate receptor antagonist) and acamprosate (a modulator of NMDA and GABA receptors) are two interventions with approval from the U.S. Food and Drug Administration (FDA) that are used in older adults to maintain sobriety from alcohol by decreasing the cravings for drinking. Naltrexone may be an excellent option for this patient. Disulfiram is not considered safe in older adults due to toxic effects.

PSYCHOTHERAPEUTIC MODALITIES

Supportive therapy and cognitive–behavioral therapy (CBT) are successful interventions for SUDs. Supportive therapies are geared toward building a trusting relation with the therapist and improving self-esteem. The clinician educates the patient about treatment principles and abstinence, explaining that the psychotropic effects of the drugs are short-lived and the substances worsen anxiety, depression, and sleep problems. CBT identifies maladaptive sequences of thoughts and behavior related to the substance use problem. These thoughts are further restructured toward positive thinking. CBT has been shown to be effective with older adults.

ALCOHOLICS/NARCOTICS ANONYMOUS (AA/NA)

AA or NA can help older adults in reducing isolation and stigma. There are a number of benefits of joining AA/NA programs, including the fact that they are readily available and free of cost. However, older individuals may face barriers to attending groups, due to shame and reluctance to disclose intimate details to younger participants. Self-help groups tailored toward older adults, allowing a slower pace and generational bonding, may overcome such difficulties.

KEY POINTS TO REMEMBER

- SUDs pose unique risks to older individuals due to the effects of aging on metabolism and the brain. Alcohol use disorder is the most common SUD in late life.
- Signs and symptoms of SUDs are important to recognize as they present in physical, psychiatric, and social dimensions. They are sometimes masked by other comorbid conditions.
- Comorbid anxiety, depression, and sleep disorders are commonly associated with SUDs and should be treated promptly, using both therapeutic approaches and standard antidepressants or other targeted medications while avoiding use of benzodiazepines.
- Treatment should address acute withdrawal states as well as maintenance approaches using medications as well as psychotherapy and support groups such as AA or NA.

Further Reading

Brown RL, Leonard T, Saunders LA, Papasouliotis O. The prevalence and detection of substance use disorder among inpatients ages 18 to 49: An opportunity for prevention. *Prev Med.* 1998;27:101–110.

Kuerbis A, Sacco P, Blazer DG, Moore AA. Substance abuse among older adults. *Clin Geriatr Med.* 2014;30(3):629–654.

Rieb LM, Samaan Z, Furlan AD, Rabheru K, Feldman S, Hung L, Budd G, Coleman D. Canadian guidelines on opioid use disorder among older adults. *Can Geriatr J.* 2020;23(1):123–134.

29 No one can work with her

Marc E. Agronin

An 88-year-old woman with a 4-year history
of progressive cognitive impairment and a
diagnosis of Alzheimer's disease is referred
to you because of increasing resistance to the
caregivers who live with her 24/7. For several
months she has had angry outbursts at several
of the aides. She sometimes refuses to eat
the food they make and throws it on the floor.
She has accused them of trying to kill her and
resists when they try to get her to take a shower
or change her clothes. She is generally calmer
and cooperative when her daughter is present
without the aides. The situation came to a crisis
one day when the woman took the aide's purse
and threw it out the front door and starting
screaming loudly. When the police arrived, she
was calmer and had no recollection of what
she did. The aide, however, was so fed up with
the woman's behavior that she quit on the
spot, leaving the daughter scrambling to get
more help.

What do you do now?

Agitation and other behavioral disturbances are common manifestations of all neurocognitive disorders (NCDs), and pose some of the most difficult and dangerous dilemmas for caregivers and clinicians. It is estimated that up to 90% of all individuals with NCDs have agitation at some point over the course of the disease. According to the International Psychogeriatric Association (IPA), agitation involves excessive motor activity, or verbal or physical aggression that causes observed (or inferred) emotional distress, and is "severe enough to produce excess disability" along with significant impairment in interpersonal relationships, social functioning, and/or the ability to perform or participate in daily living activities. A broader term that has been used is "behavioral and psychological problems of dementia" (BPSD); it includes a variety of relevant behaviors, ranging from verbal and physical agitation and aggression, to mood disturbances such as depression and anxiety, to psychosis to disinhibition. It is an important term since agitation is almost always associated with one or more of these other disturbances.

Many clinicians feel overwhelmed when a patient is highly agitated and resistant and are quick to prescribe sedating medications, but these can actually compound the situation by causing side effects. There is, however, a step-by-step approach that can clarify what is happening, identify the underlying causes, and suggest some logical courses of action. This approach is well captured by the DICE algorithm (Describe, Investigate, Create, and Evaluate) developed by Kales, Gitlin, and Lyketsos (Table 29.1).

Agitation is associated with accelerated disease progression and involves disproportionate reductions in daily function and well-being, increased healthcare utilization and costs, increased risk of injury to self and others, higher rates of institutionalization, increased mortality, and significantly worse caregiver stress and overall burden.

STEP 1: DESCRIBE

The first step is to clearly and accurately list the problematic behaviors in order to best understand what is happening, determine causes, prioritize treatments, and track progress. There are often multiple behaviors going on that need to be addressed, sometimes in sequence and other times together. It is particularly important to distinguish the phenomena from one another,

TABLE 29.1 **The DICE algorithm**

Domain	Elements
Describe	Obtain description of behaviors from caregivers. Review the context of the behaviors (when, where, with whom).
Investigate	Examine patient factors (e.g., medical and psychiatric conditions, medications), caregiver factors, environmental factors, and cultural factors.
Create	Use a team approach to respond to physical problems, develop behavioral approaches, and devise a pharmacologic approach.
Investigate	Evaluate the degree of implementation of the plan and the overall results.

especially confusion over events or people versus delusional thoughts, and misperceptions due to poor vision or illusions versus actual hallucinations. Determine the context of the behaviors, including when they occur and under what circumstances. There may be specific triggers and responses that reinforce them, such as attention-seeking agitated behaviors (e.g., screaming) set off by boredom that are gratified when others rush to engage them. Be certain to gather descriptions of the behaviors from anyone who is exposed to them and who is involved with the patient's care.

The woman's behaviors include paranoid delusions, belligerent attitudes, resistance to care, and physical aggression, including assaultiveness and destruction of property. These behaviors are mostly triggered by the presence of unfamiliar people in the house (i.e., her aides) and their attempts to provide hands-on help. They are not present with her daughter and she has no insight into them or recollection of them afterwards, which limits the ability to discuss them with her.

STEP 2: INVESTIGATE

Agitated behaviors always have a context, which includes the precipitating or causative factors as well as reactions that might serve to reinforce them. Many of the most common causative factors are listed in Table 29.2. An investigation into these factors will include close observation and interviews

TABLE 29.2 Causes of agitation

Causative factors	Examples
Medical symptoms and conditions	Delirium, metabolic imbalances, infection, trauma, pain
Medications	Stimulants, steroids, opiates, psychotropics
Psychiatric symptoms and conditions	Depression, anxiety, phobias, psychosis, sleep disorders
Psychological states	Fears, unmet needs (e.g., hunger, thirst), boredom, grief, overstimulation, poor sleep, yearning for close family, desire to escape
Environmental	Unpleasant or uncomfortable temperatures, noises, smells, lights, or sensations; inadequate or poorly skilled caregiving; lack of familiar surroundings or people; lack of structure in daily routine; lack of adequate stimulation in activities; neglect or abuse

with caregivers, medical and psychiatric exams, and laboratory and other tests. The clinician should also ask what function the behavior serves, including getting attention, escaping or avoiding something, self-stimulation, expressing something, or obtaining some tangible item (e.g., food).

An in-depth evaluation revealed ongoing pain from osteoarthritis in her back as well as a previous history of anxiety and panic attacks that were not well treated. She is more irritable when she does not sleep well or stay hydrated. Anything unfamiliar in her surroundings appears to trigger the worst of her behaviors.

STEP 3: CREATE

Once you have a clear understanding of the problematic behaviors and their context, it's time to create a treatment plan. Behavioral interventions should always be the first approach, based on knowing the person well so an individualized approach can be used. In the moment, agitated individuals can be distracted and redirected into calmer circumstances or activities. Provide for any unmet needs (e.g., hunger, thirst, toileting), and address environmental stresses (e.g., excessive noise, heat or cold, disruptive roommates). On a regular basis get the person involved in stimulating, pleasant activities such as exercise, groups, or art, music, or pet therapy. Get multiple caregivers and family members in the process.

When behaviors are resistant to behavioral interventions and pose a risk of harm to the person or others, or are causing extreme distress, pharmacologic approaches are needed. There is no universally recognized or U.S. Food and Drug Administration (FDA)-designated indication for agitation or psychosis associated with dementia, or general BPSD; thus, all psychotropic medication use is considered "off-label." Even though there has been a lot of research, clinical trials of agitation in dementia have not established significant efficacy for any psychotropic medication. In addition, many studies are of short duration; use small samples, multiple instruments, variable definitions, and limited samples; are not always controlled; and have high placebo responses. Nonetheless, there are many potential medication classes that can be used. Pros and cons are listed in Table 29.3 for some but not all of the most commonly prescribed psychotropic agents.

The woman's pain was treated with regular use of a nonsteroidal medication and physical therapy. Her anxiety and panic were treated with the selective serotonin reuptake inhibitor (SSRI) antidepressant escitalopram at 5 mg daily. She was overall calmer after a few weeks, but she was still not sleeping well or taking in enough fluids during the day. She remained anxious and paranoid about the aides and still was getting agitated on a regular basis, although with less intensity and frequency.

STEP 4: EVALUATE

Agitation and other behavioral disturbances can be challenging to improve, and may take several attempts and revisions in treatment. This is common, and requires ongoing attention to how interventions work and revising of the plan. To best evaluate progress, obtain feedback from caregivers based on multiple observations over time, since what you see during an evaluation is a single point in time and can give a misleading impression. Always be open to revising what you think is causing the behaviors, since this will, in turn, prompt logical changes in the treatment. Even if behavioral approaches don't work right away, don't forget about them in the rush to find the right

TABLE 29.3 Pros and cons of various medications for agitation

Medication class	Pros	Cons
ANTIPSYCHOTICS · Risperidone (0.25–2 mg/day) · Olanzapine (2.5–10 mg/day) · Quetiapine (25–200 mg/day) · Aripiprazole (2–10 mg/day)	· Best efficacy in studies, although benefits are modest and variable · Work best for psychotic symptoms	· Metabolic side effects · Movement disorders · Risk for cerebrovascular events and increased mortality
BENZODIAZEPINES · Lorazepam (0.25–1 mg/day) · Alprazolam (0.25–1 mg/day) · Clonazepam (0.25–1 mg/day)	· Work quickly and effectively for calming and sedation · Versatile, as-needed dosing	· Excess sedation and fall risk · Increased confusion · Paradoxical effects
ANTIDEPRESSANTS · Citalopram (10–40 mg/day) · Escitalopram (5–20 mg/day) · Sertraline (25–200 mg/day) · Mirtazapine (7.5–45 mg/day) · Venlafaxine (75–225 mg/day)	· Increasing scientific support for efficacy · Address underlying depressive and anxiety disorders · Work over time and is generally safe and well tolerated	· Take time to work (i.e., weeks) · Can sometimes increase agitation · Side effects not always tolerated
MOOD STABILIZERS · Valproic acid (250–1,000 mg/day) · Lamotrigine (2–150 mg/day)	· Best for underlying mania, bipolar disorder, or recurrent depression	· Poor efficacy in studies · Metabolic effects and drug interactions · Serum levels required for valproic acid · Risk of serious skin rash with lamotrigine

TABLE 29.3 **Continued**

Medication class	Pros	Cons
COGNITIVE ENHANCERS · Donepezil (5–10 mg/day) · Rivastigmine (6–12 mg/day for pills; 4.6–13.3 mg/day for skin patch) · Galantamine (8–16 mg/day) · Memantine (10–20 mg/day immediate release; 14–28 mg/day extended release)	· Used to boost cognition · May reduce the risk of agitation	· Poor efficacy overall and not useful in acute situations · Gastrointestinal side effects for cholinesterase inhibitors

OTHERS
Dextromethorphan + quinidine; prazosin; beta-blockers; estrogen

medication. The same evaluation process applies to medications; if one class doesn't work, try another, always thinking about matching the best medication to the most salient target symptoms. For example, psychotic symptoms require antipsychotic medications, and symptoms of depression or anxiety require antidepressants. With persistence, most behavioral disturbances yield to treatment.

After 4 weeks of partial improvement but ongoing agitation and psychosis, the escitalopram was increased to 10 mg, with additional improvement in agitation. The paranoid delusions were persistent and appeared to be major triggers, so risperidone 0.25 mg was added at bedtime, and the dose was increased to 0.5 mg after 1 week. The paranoid delusions went away after within 2 weeks and the woman began sleeping better. Her daughter brought in regular music therapy to the house, which the woman enjoyed immensely. She still refused to drink enough fluids during the day but was less resistant and hostile to the aides when they brought her meals and provided hands-on care.

- Agitation is common across all forms of dementia and is often associated with other BPSD, including anxiety, depression, and psychosis.
- A helpful algorithm to manage agitation is DICE (Describe, Investigate, Create, and Evaluate).
- The best management strategy starts with a clear understanding of the context for the behaviors, including causes and responses, and uses medical and psychiatric exams to help identify these.
- It is important to re-evaluate the treatment response and adjust the plan accordingly.

Further Reading

Cummings J, Mintzer J, Brodaty H, Sano M, Banerjee S, Devanand DP, Gauthier S, Howard R, Lanctôt K, Lyketos CG, Peskind E, Porsteinsson AP, Reich E, Sampaio C, Steffens D, Wortmann M, Zhong K; International Psychogeriatric Association. Agitation in cognitive disorders: International Psychogeriatric Association provisional consensus clinical and research definition. *Int Psychogeriatr.* 2015;27(1):7–17.

Davies SJ, Burhan AM, Kim D, Gerretsen P, Grauff-Guerrero A, Woo VL, Kumar S, Colman S, Pollock BG, Mulsant BH, Rajji TK. Sequential drug treatment algorithm for agitation and aggression in Alzheimer's and mixed dementia. *J Psychopharmacol.* 2018;32(5):509–523.

Gitlin LN, Kales HC, Lyketsos CG. Nonpharmacologic management of behavioral symptoms in dementia. *JAMA.* 2012;308(19):2020–2029.

Kales HC, Gitlin LN, Lyketsos CG; Detroit Expert Panel on Assessment and Management of Neuropsychiatric Symptoms of Dementia. Management of neuropsychiatric symptoms of dementia in clinical settings: Recommendations from a multidisciplinary expert panel. *J Am Geriatr Soc.* 2014; 62(4):762–769.

30 Trustworthy or not?

Karen Reimers

An 88-year-old recent widow is brought to your outpatient clinic by her son. She has a history of depression, generalized anxiety and a specific needle phobia. She was hospitalized twice for suicide attempts decades ago. She also has rheumatoid arthritis and type 2 diabetes. She lives alone and her son is her main support and visits a few times per month. She has been recently estranged from her two other children since a family argument. She is comfortable financially and still drives occasionally.

Her son reports that his mother recently got lost while driving. She refuses to start insulin for her diabetes due to her needle phobia. On mental status examination, she is alert and oriented to person but not place, and struggles with object recall on cognitive screening. She reports a depressed mood and struggling to find "a new normal" since her husband died.

What do you do now?

Medicolegal questions abound in geriatric psychiatry, involving federal and state laws and rules, clinical assessment and treatment issues, ethical principles, and liability/risk management factors. The patient has multiple vulnerabilities and risk factors for impaired decision-making based on the presentation and her cognitive deficits. Possible diagnoses include a neurocognitive disorder, delirium, or depression with pseudodementia. As a group, different forms of dementia (now called neurocognitive disorders [NCDs]) represent the most important reason for diminished decision-making capacity in seniors. At this point in the clinical management, screening tests to consider could include the Montreal Cognitive Assessment (MoCA), Mini–Mental State Examination (MMSE), or St. Louis University Mental Status exam (SLUMS), among several others, along with a comprehensive clinical assessment and collateral information, typically from family members. The presence of an NCD is also a significant risk factor for impaired driving, elder abuse, and financial exploitation and undue influence. Box 30.1 lists additional risk factors for impaired decision-making capacity.

The patient's family doctor contacts you with concerns about her refusal to consider insulin for her diabetes. The doctor wonders about the impact of her refusal and about her disproportionate fear of needles and injections on the treatment outcome of her diabetes, including increased risk of mortality. The doctor asks if you can help her conduct a proper assessment of the patient's decision-making, taking the relevant factors into account. You decide to investigate further into established interview questions that could help you determine whether she has capacity to refuse insulin.

BOX 30.1 **Risk factors for impaired decision-making capacity**

- Fear of or discomfort with healthcare
- Age >85 years
- Chronic neurologic condition
- Chronic psychiatric condition
- Low education level
- Significant cultural or language barrier

ASSESSMENT OF DECISION-MAKING CAPACITY

Determination of capacity is not meant to be all-encompassing and static, but rather considered specific to a situation and decision. The stringency of criteria used to assess capacity should vary according to the situation: the more serious the consequences of the decision, the more stringent the criteria for intact capacity. This is sometimes referred to as a "sliding scale" of capacity that factors in the relationship between an individual's level of cognition and the situation-specific complexity. The more complex the situation and the lower level of cognition, the greater the chance the person may lack decision-making capacity. On the other hand, the higher level of cognition and the less complicated the decision, the greater the chance that there will be decision-making capacity.

Given this sliding-scale concept of decision-making capacity, an inherent tension for many clinicians in arriving at a capacity decision is the fact that a dichotomous yes/no answer about capacity is requested in the courts or legal arena. Legal criteria for decision-making capacity about medical decisions vary depending on location and jurisdiction, but in general they include the abilities to communicate a choice, to understand the relevant information, to appreciate the medical consequences of the situation, and to reason about treatment choices. These four basic components of capacity based on Paul Appelbaum's seminal paper are summarized in Table 30.1, including practical questions to ask.

TABLE 30.1 **Criteria for medical decision-making capacity**

Component of capacity	Relevant question
Communicate a choice	Can you tell me what your decision is?
Understand the relevant information	Can you tell me in your own words about your medical condition and its treatment?
Appreciate the medical consequences of the situation	What is wrong with your health and what is treatment likely to do for you?
Reason about treatment choices	How did you decide to accept or reject the recommended treatment?

The patient reluctantly agreed to try the insulin, and told her son she would drive herself to the pharmacy to pick up the prescription. The son then expresses his concern that her driving is unsafe. In response, she argues that she has been driving for over 60 years, and currently only drives during the daytime, in good weather, not during rush hour or on highways, and less than 10 miles per week. The patient and son then consulted the doctor on what to do.

DRIVING CAPACITY

Clinicians working with older adults often find themselves in the unenviable position of needing to recommend that the patient stops driving, since this can trigger significant resistance and threaten the therapeutic alliance with the patient. Older drivers may be at greater risk for crashes due with age-related sensory or motor changes, medication effects, and neurocognitive symptoms that affect attention, decision-making, and motor and visuo-spatial skills, among others. Even though many older adult drivers like the patient in question will self-regulate their driving behavior, their own self-reports or self-assessments are not adequate measures of their fitness to drive or reliable safeguards to mitigate the risk.

An assessment of underlying functional abilities important for safe driving should determine the need for further evaluation and subsequent intervention, and for a more specialized driving evaluation. The most important functional areas for driving are summarized in Table 30.2. These key domains, along with general physical function, medical comorbidities, and medications, can help clinicians determine if a patient is at high risk for an accident and whether to recommend driving cessation.

Given the patient's high-risk status, you discuss concerns about her driving and refer her for specialized testing. She is upset, but agrees to go to a memory center that offers both computerized assessment and, if warranted, an actual driving test. Unfortunately, she fails the test and returns to your office, complaining about it. You empathize with her sadness about no longer being allowed to drive and counsel her about safety and her unwanted "retirement" from driving. She doesn't know how she will manage her weekly errands on her own. After several meetings, her son agrees to be a regular driver for her and help out with daily errands and home maintenance and cooking in exchange for some financial assistance. After some time, the patient feels increasingly

TABLE 30.2 **Important functional areas for driving**

Domain	Specific functions	Standardized Tests
Vision	· Visual acuity · Visual fields · Contrast sensitivity	· Snellen E Chart · Visual fields by confrontation testing
Cognition	· Memory · Visual perception · Processing speed · Attention · Executive function language · Insight	· Montreal Cognitive Assessment (MoCA) · Trail-Making Test, Part A and then Part B · Clock-Drawing Test · Snellgrove Maze Test
Motor/ somatosensory	· Functional range of motion · Proprioception · Endurance	· Rapid Pace Walk and/or Get Up and Go · Functional range of motion

dependent on her son and worries that she would need to move into a nursing home without his help. Her son begins helping with her personal and financial affairs, and suggests that she grant him power of attorney to better handle these matters. When you meet with the patient, she clearly has some cognitive changes, but she expresses concern about her son taking over her finances and says she feels pressured to sign documents without fully understanding them. As you listen to her description, you begin to wonder if there is an element of elder abuse.

ELDER ABUSE

Clinicians should be aware of the potential for elder abuse whenever others are heavily involved in an elder's life, either in a caregiving role or as outside agents or providers. Elder abuse can involve physical, sexual, psychological, and financial abuse and neglect. It is a large and growing problem. In the United States, at least 1 in 10 adults aged 60 and older living in their own homes experiences abuse, neglect, or exploitation annually—numbering in the millions each year. Relatively few cases of elder abuse are reported to authorities. Reasons for this include failure to recognize signs of abuse, shame about the abuse, and fear of retribution. Key risk factors for abuse among vulnerable community-dwelling older adults include physical or cognitive impairment and social isolation. Abusers often live with the vulnerable older adults, thus increasing their contact, and many suffer from mental illness or substance abuse.

Elder financial abuse is the illegal or improper use of an elder's assets, the misuse, mismanagement, or exploitation of an older person's property, belongings, or assets. This includes using an older person's assets without consent, under false justification, or via the use of intimidation and manipulation. Scams targeting elders abound, and even someone the elder has never met can steal their financial information using the telephone, internet, or email. Practical examples of elder financial exploitation include cashing an elder's social security or pension checks without permission, taking money or property from the elder, coercing or deceiving an older person into parting with property or signing documents, and diverting financial resources. Clinicians should consider the possibility of elder financial exploitation when a family caregiver wants financial control while personally being financially stressed.

The patient's daughter visits and notices that her mother's utility bills were not being paid, and that her brother had asked the mother to sign a check for $30,000 as a "loan." As a result, the daughter and her other siblings file a lawsuit against the brother alleging undue influence on the patient. It is also discovered that the son arranged for the patient to change her will, disinheriting her other two adult children and leaving her entire estate to him instead of to all three children equally as outlined in her prior will. He insists that the current arrangement is the mother's idea and in her best interest, pointing out that he cares for her and lives with her full time, whereas his siblings never visit and had been estranged from his mother for some time. As the treating psychiatrist, you are asked to provide a medical opinion in this case.

Undue influence is a legal concept by which a person is induced to act other than by their own free will. One major risk factor is having a specific person in a position of trust or upon whom the elder is dependent for emotional or physical needs, as was the case with this patient. Concerning signs might include when this person in a position of trust begins to isolate or sequester the person from other family or friends, especially in the setting of family conflict. Vulnerable older adults often suffer from a range of physical or psychological disorders that make them dependent on the trusted person, including physical or sensory disabilities, dementia, delirium, severe anxiety or depression, substance abuse, and personality disorders. Signs of tampering with the person's decision-making include sudden legal changes instigated by the beneficiary in terms of wills, insurance policies, and access to finances, especially when these changes run counter to the person's previous wishes.

The siblings' legal battle over their brother's undue influence over his mother was settled out of court. An investigation is opened through adult protective services (APS), and it emerges that the brother had been using his mother's accounts to pay for his personal expenses, depleting her savings. Eventually her accounts were secured and the patient was moved into an assisted living facility, with her personal and financial affairs being overseen by a court-appointed guardian.

KEY POINTS TO REMEMBER

- Medicolegal questions abound in geriatric psychiatry, involving federal and state laws and rules, clinical assessment and treatment issues, ethical principles, and liability/risk management factors.
- Criteria for decision-making capacity include the ability to communicate a choice, understand the relevant information, appreciate the consequences of the situation, and reason about options and alternatives.
- A variety of functional issues can influence an older patient's driving ability; clinicians may need to refer patients for specialized testing and counsel patients about "retirement" from driving.
- Elder financial exploitation, which is becoming widespread, involves the misuse, mismanagement, or exploitation of the older person's property, belongings, or assets.
- Risk factors and "red flags" for undue influence include relationship, social/environmental, psychological, physical, and legal considerations.

Further Reading

ABA/APA Assessment of Capacity in Older Adults Project Working Group. *Assessment of Older Adults with Diminished Capacity: A Handbook for Psychologists*. American Bar Association Commission on Law and Aging, American Psychological Association; 2008.

American Geriatrics Society & Pomidor A, ed. *Clinician's Guide to Assessing and Counseling Older Drivers* (4th ed.) (Report No. DOT HS 812 228.) National Highway Traffic Safety Administration, American Geriatrics Society; 2019.

Appelbaum PS. Clinical practice: Assessment of patients' competence to consent to treatment. *N Engl J Med*. 2007;357(18):1834–1840.

Barstow C, Shahan B, Roberts M. Evaluating medical decision-making capacity in practice. *Am Fam Physician*. 2018;98(1):40–46.

Peisah C, Finkel S, Shulman K, Melding P, Luxenberg J, Heinik J, Jacoby R, Reisberg B, Stoppe G, Barker A, Firmino H, Bennett H; International Psychogeriatric Association Task Force on Wills and Undue Influence. The wills of older people: Risk factors for undue influence. *Int Psychogeriatr*. 2009;21(1):7–15.

Shulman KI, Cohen CA, Kirsh FC, Hull IM, Champine PR. Assessment of testamentary capacity and vulnerability to undue influence. *Am J Psychiatry*. 2007;164(5):722–727.

31 Wired and ready

Kathryn Kieran and Ipsit V. Vahia

A 70-year-old widowed, female is referred
for geriatric psychiatry evaluation by her
primary care physician (PCP) with diagnoses
of mild cognitive impairment (MCI) and
major depressive disorder (MDD). Her history
includes one psychiatric hospitalization after an
unintentional overdose in the preceding year.
She lives alone with part time caregiver help and
her daughter drives 2 hours to fill her medication
organizer on weekends. She occasionally uses
her home desktop computer and a smartphone
but acknowledges that she does not know how
to use most features on her phone.

Medically she has diagnoses of psoriasis and
asthma that is exacerbated in winter. Her medication
list consists of lorazepam, fluoxetine, albuterol inhaler,
and topical steroid cream. She is very motivated to
establish care over audiovisual telehealth, but "I don't
know where to begin."

What do you do now?

This case raises several key questions with respect to introducing technology-naïve patients to telecare and digital mental health: How would you assess for tech-readiness in this patient? Would you encourage or discourage particular technological solutions? And finally, how would you create an inventory of resources for success?

GETTING PATIENTS TECH-READY

A patient-centered discussion of initiating digital care must begin with collecting an inventory of what devices or technology the patient currently owns and assessing their access and proficiency in using the internet and internet-based services (e.g., email, social media). It is also important to gauge their interest and capability around learning the use of digital tools. Factors such as cognitive impairment, deficits in fine motor function, or neurologic symptoms such as tremors may need to be taken into account. As such, tablet devices have been found to be most user-friendly for older adults. If the patient does not already have email access, selecting one must be the priority, so invitations to appointments and registrations for devices, apps, and other functionality can be completed. Equipment availability can guide some recommendations. A desktop computer like the one our patient has may need a webcam to enable audiovisual telehealth visits. Broadly speaking, laptops and tablet-style home computers are easier to manipulate and use than a smartphone, as higher levels of finger dexterity are required for the smaller and closer-together icons and buttons. Patients in crowded environments may prefer headphones with an integrated microphone, for increased privacy. Encouraging patients to always wear any assistive devices to appointments, such as hearing aids, dentures, and visual aids, will facilitate effective two-way communication.

When feasible, a trial run of an appointment with clinic staff should be encouraged. If an organization's support staff or patient supports are available to assist the patient in setting up technology and training them in optimal use, their assistance is invaluable. Studies have shown that older adults living in households with multiple generations tend to be more proficient at using various technologies. For patients in assisted living facilities, facility staff may also be able to help. When possible, scheduling appointments so more technologically savvy friends, family, or other caregivers can be available is recommended. An important caveat: Interpersonal dynamics may be more complicated than they first appear. Best practice remains that a part of the appointment is solely with the patient in the room to share any personal concerns they would rather not share with others, including past or present abuse or neglect, sexual health, issues of identity, and so forth.

MOTIVATING SUCCESSFUL USE

Successful use of technology is most likely if clinicians serve as advocates for the technology and are proficient in its use, existing technology is optimized, and sufficient time and effort is spent in training older adults to use the selected technology appropriately. In addition, it is important to note that while older adults tend to use technology in a more targeted and individualized manner, if appropriately trained and if the technology meets a perceived need to enhance care, rates of adherence to technology-based interventions among older adults are higher than those among younger adults. This holds true for telemedicine but also apps, wearables, or other sensors.

COMMUNICATION TECHNOLOGIES

The advent of the COVID-19 pandemic in the spring of 2020 led to massive adoption of numerous telemedicine platforms. This was a global phenomenon, and at the time of writing, we are still in the process of understanding what types of care may be best delivered via telemedicine versus traditional in-person care. When selecting communication technologies, clinicians must be cognizant of the platform in use. While commercial tools such as Skype or FaceTime may be more convenient, security features can be underdeveloped, and there is a risk of compromising patient privacy. Many healthcare systems have adopted platforms that are compliant with the Health Insurance Portability and Accountability Act (HIPAA), and these are preferable. Most platforms can be used over a range of devices, including smartphones, tablets, and computers. Older adults should be encouraged to communicate using the device that is easiest for them to use. When choice is available, a desktop or a laptop on a stable surface, as our patient has at home, may be preferable.

APPS AND PROGRAMS

Once the appropriate hardware is available and functional, compatible apps and programs can be suggested. Finding reliable, safe medical devices and software to recommend can be a challenge, given the broad variety flooding the market, and the lack of regulation. In general, apps can be classified into three broad categories: communication apps, technologies for assessment and monitoring, and technologies for delivering interventions (sometimes referred to as digital therapeutics). The U.S. Food and Drug Administration (FDA) is continuing development of an oversight program, currently in pilot phase, called the Digital Software Pre-Cert Program (https://www.fda.gov/medical-devices/digital-hea lth-software-precertification-pre-cert-program/precertification-pre-cert-pilot-program-frequently-asked-questions). The U.S. Department of Veterans Affairs has "coach" apps, including for sleep, PTSD, and relationships, that are available in an online "store" to any user (https://mobile.va.gov/appstore/mental-health).

Many attempts have been made to develop app-rating systems, but none has attained ascendency, or had the resources to continually update and refine any kind of comprehensive database. The American Psychiatric Association (APA) has developed an alternative app-evaluation model called the App Advisor (https://www.psychiatry.org/psychiatrists/pract ice/mental-health-apps/the-app-evaluation-model)with five levels of questions the patient and provider can investigate before using an app. This approach provides clinicians and patients a framework by which they can assess any app independently. Safety and privacy concerns precede all other considerations, as data mining and targeting older adults for scams are real risks.

A major challenge with the use of apps for mental health is a relative lack of evidence to support their efficacy. There are few well-designed clinical trials assessing the efficacy and effectiveness of mental health apps to date. One indication that appears to be well supported is mindfulness. More specific treatments such as cognitive–behavioral therapy, acceptance and commitment therapy, or other specific modality apps may be more selectively recommended. Studies to date indicate that such apps are most effective when they are used to support, rather than replace, an actual therapist. Many mood-monitoring apps can provide a high degree of longitudinal data and store these data for review during session. Other apps may also serve to organize medications or keep track of appointments. A small number of apps developed by specific healthcare systems provide secure closed channels for patients to communicate with their providers. However, the use of these varies greatly depending on clinical setting and geographic location. It is also important for clinicians to gauge the utility of recommending a widely used commercial app that may potentially impact the patient's lifestyle and independence. Examples of this include ride-sharing apps, which may provide transportation and reduce the need for driving, or food-delivery apps, which provide an easier alternative to cooking. *In our patient, both of these examples may be applicable in order to reduce costs to the family and time and travel for the patient's daughter.*

WEARABLES

Wearable devices such as fitness monitors and smartwatches can provide heart rate and sleep information that can greatly assist the clinician when making medication adjustments. Current wearable technology can track and monitor motion, which in turn can be used for a wide range of indications, including monitoring sleep, physical activity, and inert time. While these are generally lifestyle enhancement devices, the data they collect can be leveraged to monitor psychiatrically relevant clinical parameters. Increasingly, wearable devices are also able to capture vital signs such as heart rate, oxygen saturation, and temperature. Efforts are under way to create a blood pressure (B) monitor that is effective through a wearable like a watch, without the need for compression. Many patients already have BP monitors at home and can take a reading right in front of you during appointments, and many at-home BP monitors store information that can be recalled and shared via phone calls, messaging in the integrated electronic health record (EHR), or email. Titration of sleep and anxiety medication can be guided in part by this data, along with collateral information, if the patient's self-report is inconsistent. A note of caution: Not all wearables have sensors that have been tested on a wide range of skin tones, and this must be considered when researching and recommending these technologies.

PASSIVE SENSING, AND THE ADVENT OF TOOLS SUPPORTED BY ARTIFICIAL INTELLIGENCE (AI)

Because of extraordinary advancements in sensor technologies, a broad range of in-home devices can be leveraged to support geriatric mental health care. A common example is voice-activated smart home technologies such as the Amazon Echo or Google Home. These devices are supported by AI and respond to voice commands. Early evidence suggests that this technology can support older adults living independently with cognitive challenges. In addition to these integrated devices, a wide range of sensor-equipped tools such as bathroom scales now have app integration and can send information to providers, but a lower-tech option is taking a reading during an appointment and showing the result on the screen. Other AI-based approaches like natural language processing are also in the early stages of study for use with older adults. For instance, this technology can aggregate language in the texts, emails, and social media content the patient creates. When assessing cognition, this information, reviewed always with the patient's informed consent, may provide real-time examples of episodes of confusion, language skills, and the status of instrumental activities of daily living such as ordering groceries or food takeout. They can also provide insights into changes in personality and interpersonal functioning, as when a disagreement with a partner or family member is stored in text form. Interpersonal interactions can also provide important fodder for mentalizing practice and challenging cognitive distortions. *For our patient, use of a voice-assisted technology for appointment and medication reminders could help to reduce caregiver role strain.*

ASSESSING RISK AND TROUBLESHOOTING

Any use of technology must be centered around clinical indication and patient preferences. It should also be grounded in the patient's own history. Trauma-informed care remains crucial and should include offering choices at every opportunity. Inquiry about trauma upon establishing care should be focused on its effects on current functioning. Some patients will share experiences of audiovisual trauma, voyeurism, and other forms of harm from being watched or recorded. The activation of paranoid ideation is also important to consider, especially if deploying a technology for monitoring. At times the patient can articulate a specific aversive aspect of the telehealth experience, such as viewing themselves on the screen. Many telehealth platforms allow patients to hide themselves from view during a session. Other sources of discomfort have low-tech solutions, such as a red light near the camera reminding them of a traumatic recording experience; the light can be covered with a small piece of opaque tape. *Given our patient's history of trauma, any requests of this nature should be honored wherever possible.*

CAREGIVER CONCERNS

Caregivers may also have questions about technology to help them monitor their loved one's health status from afar. There are a variety of tools on the market that will dispense medications at predetermined times to reduce medication errors. Some services will monitor doorways for entrance and exit or send the patient's GPS location in case of wandering. There are even robots programmed to attempt to reduce social isolation through simulated interaction as well as programmed reminders for medications, activities of daily living, and appointments. Motion mapping and other emerging technologies will make safety monitoring increasingly unobtrusive. In resource-rich and time-poor environments, these measures may be within reach. Patients without internet access at home, on the other hand, can make use of community hotspots, courses, and sometimes live tech support at or near libraries and senior centers.

KEY POINTS TO REMEMBER

- Equipment and readiness assessment will guide next steps.
- Help from aides, family, friends, and community resources may be called upon.
- Apps can be evaluated, even if a database of reliable apps does not yet exist; the source should always be considered.
- Trauma-informed care prioritizes privacy, openness to hearing about past negative experiences, and asking about ways to make the telehealth experience more comfortable where possible.

Further Reading

Carlo AD, Hosseini Ghomi R, Renn BN, Areán PA. By the numbers: Ratings and utilization of behavioral health mobile applications. *NPJ Digit Med.* 2019;2:54.

Fortuna KL, Torous J, Depp CA, Jimenez DE, Areán PA, Walker R, Ajilore O, Goldstein CM, Cosco TD, Brooks JM, Vahia IV, Bartels SJ. A future research agenda for digital geriatric mental healthcare. *Am J Geriatr Psychiatry.* 2019;27:1277–1285.

Gould CE, Hantke NC. Promoting technology and virtual visits to improve older adult mental health in the face of COVID-19. *Am J Geriatr Psychiatry.* 2020;28:889–890.

Vahia IV, Forester BP. Motion mapping in humans as a biomarker for psychiatric disorders. *Neuropsychopharmacology.* 2019;44(1):231–232.

Index

For the benefit of digital users, indexed terms that span two pages (e.g., 52–53) may, on occasion, appear on only one of those pages.

Tables are indicated by *t* following the page number.

6-Item Screen, 39*t*

AA (Alcoholics Anonymous), 264
abnormal movements, 26*t*
absolute contraindications, 49
abuse, 259. *See also* elder abuse
acamprosate, 264
acetaminophen, 21
acetylcholinesterase inhibitors (AChEIs),
   47, 80–81, 93, 98
activities of daily living (ADLs), 11, 42*t*,
   83, 252
acute withdrawal, 263
AD. *See* Alzheimer's disease
addiction, 259
ADHD (attention-deficit/hyperactivity
   disorder), 106–7
adherence, 7
ADLs (activities of daily living), 11, 42*t*,
   83, 252
Adult Protective Services (APS), 111
adverse childhood events, 236–37
AES (Apathy Evaluation Scale), 204–5
affect, 26*t*, 29
African Americans, 90, 221
agitation, 28, 84, 267–74
   creating treatment plan, 270–71
   describing, 268–69
   with DLB, 99
   evaluating progress, 271–73
   investigating, 269–70
   overview, 268
AI (artificial intelligence), 288
AIT (Amyloid Imaging Task Force), 51–52
Alcoholics Anonymous (AA), 264

alcohol use disorder, 21, 169, 187, 216
alertness, 26*t*, 31
algorithms, treatment, 172, 173*t*
allergies, 7–8
Alzheimer's Association, 51
Alzheimer's disease, 19, 79–87
   biomarkers for diagnosing, 46–47
   clinical insights for differential
      diagnosis, 66*t*
   delusional disorder and risk of, 238
   early and mild stage, 80–83
   middle- to late-stage, moderate to
      severe, 83–85
   neurologic assessment, 16–17
   psychosis in, 221
   treatments, 85–86
American Academy of Neurology, 46–
   48, 73
American Psychiatric Association, 46–
   47, 286
amnestic MCI, 73
amyloid beta (Aß), 46–47, 86
Amyloid Imaging Task Force (AIT), 51–52
amyloid PET, 46–47, 51–52
ANA (antinuclear antibodies), 22
analgesics, 61*t*
anomia, 17–19
anosmia, 16–17
anticholinergics, 61*t*, 74, 252
antidepressants, 132–33, 141
   for agitation, 272*t*
   for delusional disorder, 238
   for depression, 174–75
   FTT and, 200
   for OCD, 150–51

antiepileptic medication levels, 22
antinuclear antibodies (ANA), 22
antipsychotics, 99, 112, 141, 224–25
    for agitation, 272t
    for delirium, 253–54
    for OCD, 150–51
    for PDP, 230–31
    with schizophrenia, 242–43
anxiety disorders, 125–33
    causes and comorbidities, 126–27
    causing MCI, 74
    with comorbid depression, 129
    due to other medical conditions, 129
    generalized anxiety disorder
        (GAD), 127–28
    medical treatments and, 130
    obsessive–compulsive disorder
        (OCD), 145–52
    panic disorder (PD), 135–43
    post-traumatic stress disorder
        (PTSD), 155–62
    prevalence of, 126
    in setting of neurodegenerative
        disorders, 128
    symptomatic anxiety
        treatment, 131–33
apathy, 203–7
    assessment, 204–5
    treatment, 205–7
    with VaD, 91
Apathy Evaluation Scale (AES), 204–5
ApoE-4 gene, 52, 64, 74
App Advisor, 286
appearance, 26t, 27–28
appropriateness, mood, 29
apps, 286–87
apraxia, 20–21
APS (Adult Protective Services), 111
artificial intelligence (AI), 288
Asians, 90
Aß (amyloid beta), 46–47, 86
ataxia, 260
atrophy, patterns of, 50
attention, 26t, 31, 42t

attention-deficit/hyperactivity disorder
    (ADHD), 106–7
attitude, 26t, 28
atypical antipsychotics, 238
augmentation, 174–75
autism spectrum disorder, 106–7
autoimmune disorders, 21, 22, 59t, 215

B12 vitamin (cobalamin), 21, 216
Babinski's sign, 19
BAL (blood alcohol level), 261
balance, 18t, 20
barium sulfate–based compounds, 48–49
Beck Anxiety Index (BAI), 74
Beers Criteria, 7, 74, 168–69
behavior, 26t, 28
behavioral and psychological problems of
    dementia (BPSD), 268, 271
behavioral variant FTD (bvFTD), 104–6,
    105t, 108t
benzodiazepines, 100, 132, 141–42,
    142t, 160–61
    for agitation, 272t
    toxicity, 258, 259–60, 261–62
    withdrawal, 263
Binswanger's disease, 90
biomarkers, 46–47, 97–98
bipolar disorder, 179–84
bleeding, 47
blood alcohol level (BAL), 261
blood levels, 180–81, 261
blood panel, 75
body mass index (BMI), 81
BPSD (behavioral and psychological
    problems of dementia), 268, 271
bradykinesia, 96
bradyphrenia, 29–30
bradypsychia, 29–30
Brief Psychiatric Rating Scale
    (BPRS), 230–31
Broca's area, 17–19
Brownian motion, 47–48
bvFTD (behavioral variant FTD), 104–6,
    105t, 108t

CAGE-AID questionnaire, 261
CAM (Confusion Assessment Method), 250
cancer, 127, 130
cannabis, 252–53, 258, 262
carbohydrate deficient transferrin (CDT), 261
cardiopulmonary complications, 136–37
cardiovascular conditions, 130*t*
cardiovascular system, 17*t*
caregivers
    communicating with, 11–12
    elder abuse, 279–81
    technology, concerns with, 289
category fluency, 39*t*
CBC (complete blood count), 21, 75, 197
CBSST (Cognitive Behavior Social Skills Therapy), 237
CBT. *See* cognitive-behavioral therapy
CBT-P (Cognitive Behavior Therapy for Psychosis), 237–38
CDT (carbohydrate deficient transferrin), 261
Center for Epidemiological Studies Depression Scale (CES-D), 74
cerebrospinal fluid, 22, 46–47
    with MRI imaging modalities, 47–48
    NPH evaluation, 118–19
Charles Bonnet syndrome, 30–31
childhood events, adverse, 236–37
cholinesterase inhibitors, 224–25, 231
cingulate island sign, 50
circumstantiality, 29–30
CJD (Creutzfeldt–Jakob disease), 22, 50
claustrophobia, 47, 49
clock drawing test (CLOX), 32–33, 39*t*
clonazepam, 100
CMP (comprehensive metabolic panel), 21
cobalamin (B12 vitamin), 21, 216
cognitive-behavioral therapy, 139*t*, 159–60, 172
    for anxiety, 132
    panic disorder (PD), 138
    for SUDs, 264

Cognitive Behavior Social Skills Therapy (CBSST), 237
Cognitive Behavior Therapy for Psychosis (CBT-P), 237–38
cognitive enhancers, 272*t*
cognitive functioning, 26*t*, 31–33
    depression and status of, 169–70
    for driving capacity, 279*t*
    dysfunction in cognitive domains, 60–65
    HPI revealing, 6*t*
    schizophrenia and deficits with, 243–44
cognitive processing therapy (CPT), 159–60
cognitive reserve, 38, 243–44
cognitive screenings, 37–44
cognitive therapy (CT), 148–49
Columbia Suicide Severity Rating Scale (C-SSRS), 171–72, 189
combination therapy, 85
communication, 4, 285
comorbidities
    anxiety disorders, 126–27, 129
    depression, 169–71
    normal pressure hydrocephalus (NPH), 120
complete blood count (CBC), 21, 75, 197
complex attention, 62*t*
comprehension, 17–19
comprehensive metabolic panel (CMP), 21
computed tomography (CT), 47–49, 90
concentration, 26*t*, 31, 42*t*
Confusion Assessment Method (CAM), 250
congenital illness, 59*t*
congruence, mood, 29
constitutional system, 17*t*
continuous performance test, 32–33
continuous positive airway pressure (CPAP), 74, 92–93
contrast brain imaging, 48–49
cooperation, 28
coordination, 18*t*, 20

Cornell Scale of Depression in Dementia (CSDD), 58, 171, 189
corticobasal syndrome, 104
COVID-19 (SARS CoV-2) virus and pandemic, 255, 285
CPAP (continuous positive airway pressure), 74, 92–93
CPT (cognitive processing therapy), 159–60
cranial nerves, 16–17, 18t
C-reactive protein (CRP), 21, 250–51
creatine phosphokinase (CPK), 21
Creutzfeldt–Jakob disease (CJD), 22, 50
crystallized intelligence, 72
CSDD (Cornell Scale of Depression in Dementia), 58, 171, 189
CSF. See cerebrospinal fluid
C-SSRS (Columbia Suicide Severity Rating Scale), 171–72, 189
CT (cognitive therapy), 148–49
CT (computed tomography), 47–49, 90

DaTscan (GE Healthcare), 53, 97
decision-making capacity, 277–78
degenerative illness, 59t
delirium, 206, 249–56, 263
delusional disorder, 233–39
delusions, 30, 96–97, 212
dementia
    delirium and, 255
    diagnosis with biomarkers and neuroimaging and, 46–47
    subtype and staging, 65
dementia with Lewy bodies, 31, 95–101
    clinical insights for differential diagnosis, 66t
    neurologic assessment, 16–17
    overview, 96–98
    pattern of atrophy, 50
    psychosis in, 222, 223t
    treatment, 98–101
dependence, 259
depression, 167–76
    assessment, 171–72

management of, 176
medical and psychiatric comorbidities, 169–71
memory loss with, 38–40
speech and, 28
substance abuse due to self-medicating for, 262
treatment, 172–75
vascular depression, 91
DESH (disproportionately enlarged subarachnoid space hydrocephalus), 117
detoxification, 260–61t
Dexedrine, 206
diagnosis
    delirium, 250–51
    delusional disorder, 236–37
    frontotemporal dementia (FTD), 106–10
    neurocognitive disorders, 58–60
    normal pressure hydrocephalus (NPH), 117–19
    obsessive–compulsive disorder (OCD), 147–48
    substance use disorders (SUDs), 260–62
    vascular dementia (VaD), 90–92
Diagnostic and Statistical Manual of Mental Disorders (DSM-5), 46–47, 104–6, 146, 156t, 158, 259
DICE algorithm, 268–73
diet, 75–76, 92–93
differential vulnerability hypothesis, 159
diffusion-weighted imaging (DWI), 47–48, 48t
Digital Software Pre-Cert Program, 286
Dimensional Obsessive-Compulsive Scale (DOCS), 146
disability, 187, 188t
disproportionately enlarged subarachnoid space hydrocephalus (DESH), 117
dissociative symptoms, 156–58
DLB. See dementia with Lewy bodies
donepezil, 81, 82t, 85, 93

dopamine agonists, 98, 99
dopaminergic medications, 61*t*,
    112, 228–29
dosing, 7
driving capacity, 43–44, 100–1, 278–79
drugs, 59*t*, 60
DSM-5 (*Diagnostic and Statistical Manual
    of Mental Disorders*), 46–47, 104–6,
    146, 156*t*, 158, 259
D vitamin level, 21
DWI (diffusion-weighted imaging),
    47–48, 48*t*
dysdiadochokinesia, 20
dysfunction in cognitive domains, 60–65

early-onset schizophrenia, 242
educational attainment, 38–40
elder abuse, 111, 279–81
electrocardiogram (ECG), 21
electroconvulsive therapy (ECT), 175,
    200–1, 231
EMDR (Eye Movement Desensitization
    and Reprocessing), 159–60
emotional function, 42*t*
empathy, 4, 9–10
encephalitides, 215*t*
encoding, 32
endocrine disorders, 59*t*, 130*t*, 214
epidemiology, delirium, 251–53
ERP (exposure and response
    prevention), 148–49
erythrocyte sedimentation rate (ESR),
    21, 250–51
ethyl glucuronide (EtG), 21
etiology, underlying, 253
Evans Index, 117
executive function, 26*t*, 32–33, 42*t*, 62*t*
exercise, 81–83
exposure and response prevention
    (ERP), 148–49
exposure therapy, 159–60
expressive language, 32
Eye Movement Desensitization and
    Reprocessing (EMDR), 159–60

failure to thrive (FTT), 195–202
falls, 260
family history, 8–9
fasciculations, 19
FAST (Functional Assessment Scale), 65
fasting lipid panel, 21
FDA (Food and Drug Administration), 76,
    80, 231, 264, 286
FDG (fluorodeoxyglucose) PET, 50–
    51, 110
financial abuse, elder, 280
finger-to-nose testing, 20
firearms, 188*t*
FLAIR, 47–48, 48*t*
fluent aphasias, 17–19
fluid intelligence, 72
fluorescent treponemal antibody absorption
    (FTAABS), 21–22
fluorodeoxyglucose (FDG) PET, 50–
    51, 110
folate, 21
folic acid deficiency, 216
Food and Drug Administration (FDA), 76,
    80, 231, 264, 286
frailty, 196*t*, 252
frontal gait disorder, 20
frontal lobe function, 20–21
frontal pathology, 19
frontal release signs, 26*t*
frontotemporal dementia (FTD), 19, 103–13
    clinical insights for differential
        diagnosis, 66*t*
    diagnosis, 106–10
    overview, 104–6
    pattern of atrophy, 50
    psychosis in, 222, 223*t*
    treatment, 110–12
FTAABS (fluorescent treponemal antibody
    absorption), 21–22
FTD motor neuron disease, 104
FTT (failure to thrive), 195–202
functional assessment, 11, 252
Functional Assessment Scale (FAST), 65
fund of knowledge, 26*t*, 32

GAD (generalized anxiety disorder), 126, 127–28
GAD-7 (General Anxiety Disorder 7-item Scale), 74
gadolinium, 48–49, 48t
gait, 18t, 20, 26t, 59, 116–17
galantamine, 81, 82t, 93
gamma-glutamyl transferase (GGT), 21, 261
gastrointestinal system, 17t, 130t
GE Healthcare (DaTscan), 53, 97
General Anxiety Disorder 7-item Scale (GAD-7), 74
generalized anxiety disorder (GAD), 126, 127–28
gene testing, 64, 110
genitourinary system, 17t
Geriatric Depression Scale (GDS), 58, 171, 189, 205
GGT (gamma-glutamyl transferase), 21, 261
global cerebral atrophy, 50
global cognitive function, 42t
glucocorticoids, 61t
glutamate, 84
glycated hemoglobin (HbA1c) level, 21

hallucinations, 30–31, 53, 96–97, 99, 212
Hamilton Depression Rating Scale (HAM-D), 189, 235–36
HbA1c (glycated hemoglobin) level, 21
Health Insurance Portability and Accountability Act (HIPAA), 285
hearing, 16–17
heavy metal screen, 22
HEENT, 17t
hepatic encephalopathy, 213–14
history of present illness (HPI), 5, 6t, 234–35
hospice care, 254–55
hospitalization, 217, 237–38
human immunodeficiency virus (HIV), 21–22
hydrocephalus ex vacuo, 117

hyperactive delirium, 254–55
hyperparathyroidism, 182
hypoactive delirium, 250
hypometabolism, 50–51
hypothyroidism, 60

iatrogenic illness, 59t
ICD-10 (International Statistical Classification of Disease and Related Health Problems), 259
idiopathic PD, 97–98
illicit substance use, 258
illusions, 30–31
immunologic conditions, 130t
immunotherapy, 86
Impact of Events Scale–Revised, 158
incontinence, 116–17, 120
infectious diseases, 21, 59t, 214–15
inflammatory disorders, 215
inoculation hypothesis, 159
insight, 26t, 33
insomnia, 74, 170, 173–74, 216, 262–63
instrumental ADLs, 11, 83
integumentary system, 17t
intensity, mood, 29
International Psychogeriatric Association (IPA), 268
International Statistical Classification of Disease and Related Health Problems (ICD-10), 259
International Workgroup Guidelines, 46–47
interoceptive sensations, 137–38
interpersonal therapy (IPT), 172
interpreters, 12
iodine, 48–49
iodine 123 ioflupane SPECT, 53
IPA (International Psychogeriatric Association), 268

judgment, 26t, 33–34

ketamine, 175
Korsakoff syndrome, 260

laboratory tests, 21–22
language, 26t, 32, 38, 42t, 62t
large-vessel disease, 91
late-life depression (LLD), 168. *See also*
    depression
later-onset schizophrenia, 242
learning, 42t, 62t
levodopa, 98, 99
Lilliputian hallucinations, 31
lithium therapy, 179–84
logopenic PPA, 19, 104, 105t
Longitudinal Aging Study Amsterdam, 126
Luria test, 20–21

magnetic metal, 49
magnetic resonance imaging (MRI), 46–
    50, 75, 90
maintenance treatment, 264
major depressive disorder (MDD), 127–28,
    158, 186–87, 236–37
major neurocognitive disorder (MNCD).
    See dementia
malnutrition, 252
MBCT (mindfulness-based cognitive
    therapy), 149
MCI. *See* mild cognitive impairment
medial temporal lobe (MTL)
    atrophy, 47, 50
medical conditions
    anxiety disorders due to other, 129
    delirium occurring with, 251–52
    increased rate of suicide with, 187
medications
    acetylcholinesterase inhibitors
        (AChEIs), 80–81
    for agitation, 272t
    associated with anxiety, 130, 131t
    exacerbating DLB symptoms, 100
    interfering with cognitive function, 74
    psychiatric history-taking, 7–8
    psychosis and, 216–17
    for PTSD, 161t
    triggering delirium, 252–53
medicolegal questions, 275–81

melatonin, 100
memantine, 84–85, 85t, 93
memory, 26t, 32, 42t, 62t
mental status examination (MSE), 5, 25–
    34, 26t, 229, 235–36
metabolic disorders, 59t, 130t, 214
metabolism, 50–51
metal, magnetic, 49
methylphenidate, 206
mild cognitive impairment, 60–64, 71–77
    assessment, 75
    risk factors and causes, 73–74
    subtypes, 73
    treatment, 75–76
mindfulness-based cognitive therapy
    (MBCT), 149
Mini-Cog test, 39t
Mini–Mental State Examination (MMSE),
    31, 39t, 61, 75, 169–70
monitoring delirium, 254
Montreal Cognitive Assessment (MoCA),
    31, 39t, 61, 75, 169–70
mood, 26t, 29, 42t
mood disorders
    apathy, 203–7
    bipolar disorder and lithium
        therapy, 179–84
    causing MCI, 74
    depression, 167–76
    failure to thrive (FTT), 195–202
    suicide, 185–92
mood stabilizers, 272t
morbidity and mortality,
    schizophrenia, 244–45
motor exam, 18t, 19, 26t
MRI (magnetic resonance imaging), 46–
    50, 75, 90
MSE (mental status examination), 5, 25–
    34, 26t, 229, 235–36
MTL (medial temporal lobe)
    atrophy, 47, 50
multidisciplinary team, 199t
multidomain MCI, 73
multifactorial geriatric syndromes, 196

muscle tone and strength, 26*t*
musculoskeletal system, 17*t*

naltrexone, 264
naming, 17–19
Narcotics Anonymous (NA), 264
National Comorbidity Survey Replication
    (NCS-R), 126
National Institute of Mental Health
    (NIMH), 230
National Institute of Neurological Disorders
    and Stroke (NINDS), 90, 230
National Institute on Aging/Alzheimer's
    Association (NIA-AA), 46–47, 52
National Survey on Drug Use and
    Health, 258
natural health products, 61*t*, 85–86
neoplasm illness, 59*t*
neurocognitive disorders (NCDs), 57–65
    agitation, 267–74
    Alzheimer's disease (AD), 79–87
    dementia subtype and staging, 65
    dementia with Lewy bodies
        (DLB), 95–101
    diagnosis, 58–60
    drugs, 60
    dysfunction in cognitive domains, 60–65
    frontotemporal dementia
        (FTD), 103–13
    mild cognitive impairment
        (MCI), 71–77
    normal pressure hydrocephalus
        (NPH), 115–21
    psychosis in, 222
    vascular dementia (VaD), 89–94
neurodegenerative disorders
    anxiety disorders in setting of, 128
    psychosis, 215–16
neuroimaging, 22, 45–54
    amyloid PET, 51–52
    bvFTD diagnosis with, 110
    dementia diagnosis with biomarkers
        and, 46–47
    fluorodeoxyglucose (FDG) PET, 50–51

with FTT, 197
for NPH diagnosis, 117
for psychosis, 212–13
SPECT, 53–54
structural imaging, 47–50
tau PET, 52–53
for VaD, 91
neurologic exam, 15–23
    gait, posture, balance, and
        coordination, 20
    laboratory tests, 21–22
    motor and sensory exam, 19
    neurologic assessment, 16–17
    speech, 17–19
    tests specific to frontal lobe
        function, 20–21
    vitals and physical exam, 16, 17*t*
neuropsychological evaluation, 40–44
neurosyphilis, 21–22
NIA-AA (National Institute on Aging/
    Alzheimer's Association), 46–47, 52
nightmares, 81, 97
NIMH (National Institute of Mental
    Health), 230
NINDS (National Institute of
    Neurological Disorders and
    Stroke), 90, 230
NMDA antagonists, 84
non-amnestic MCI, 73
non-contrast brain imaging, 48–49
nonfluent aphasia, 17–19
nonfluent PPA, 19, 104, 105*t*
nonsteroidal anti-inflammatory drugs
    (NSAIDs), 174–75
normal pressure hydrocephalus
    (NPH), 115–21

obsessive–compulsive disorder (OCD),
    106–7, 126, 145–52
obstructive sleep apnea (OSA), 74, 170
occupational therapy, 81–83
open-ended questions, 5
open MRI, 49
opiates, 142, 258, 262, 263

orientation, 26*t*, 31

pain, 170
panic disorder (PD), 126, 135–43
paraneoplastic antibodies, 22
paranoid personality, 236–37
paraphasias, 17–19
parathyroid hormone (PTH), 181
paratonia, 19
parkinsonian symptoms, 53, 59, 96
Parkinson's disease (PD), 16–17, 20,
    222, 223*t*
Parkinson's disease dementia (PDD),
    66*t*, 97–98
Parkinson's disease psychosis
    (PDP), 227–32
past medical history, 5–7, 234–35
past psychiatric history, 8
Patient Health Questionnaire (PHQ-9),
    58, 74, 171, 189
patterns of atrophy, 50
paucity of speech, 17–19
PD (panic disorder), 126, 135–43
PD (Parkinson's disease), 16–17, 20,
    222, 223*t*
PDD (Parkinson's disease dementia),
    66*t*, 97–98
PDP (Parkinson's disease
    psychosis), 227–32
perceptual disturbances, 26*t*, 30–31
perceptual-motor cognition, 62*t*
perseveration, 20–21
pharmacotherapy, 132–33, 150*t*, 160–61
phobic disorder, 126
PHQ-9 (Patient Health Questionnaire),
    58, 74, 171, 189
physical exam, 16, 17*t*
pimavanserin, 99, 231
polypharmacy, 150–51, 168, 175, 180–
    81, 253
polysomnography (PSG), 97
porphyrias, 214
post-traumatic stress disorder
    (PTSD), 155–62

posture, 18*t*, 20
Primary Care PTSD Screen, 158
primary progressive aphasia (PPA), 19, 104
problem-solving therapy (PST), 172
processing speed, 42*t*
programs, 286–87
progressive supranuclear palsy
    syndrome, 104
prostate enlargement, 120
pseudodementia, 58
PSG (polysomnography), 97
PST (problem-solving therapy), 172
psychiatric history-taking, 3–14
psychoeducation, 132, 160, 172, 237
psychomotor functioning, 42*t*
psychopharmacology, 140–43
psychosis, 205–7, 219–26
    in Alzheimer's disease (AD), 221
    causes of, 206, 213
    delusional disorder, 233–39
    in DLB, 96, 99
    memantine and, 84
    in other neurocognitive disorders
        (NCDs), 222
    overview, 204–6
    Parkinson's disease psychosis
        (PDP), 227–32
    schizophrenia, 241–46
    symptoms, 220–21
    treatment, 224–26
psychotherapy
    for AD, 81–83
    for delusional disorder, 237
    for PTSD, 159–60
    substance use disorders (SUDs), 264
    symptomatic anxiety treatment, 132
psychotropic medications, 22, 253–54
PTH (parathyroid hormone), 181
PTSD (post-traumatic stress
    disorder), 155–62
PTSD CheckList–Civilian Version, 158
pulmonary system, 17*t*
pulse oximetry, 16
putamen, 53

range, mood, 29
rapid plasma reagin (RPR), 21–22
RBD (REM sleep behavior disorder),
    97, 99–100
reactivity, mood, 29
receptive language, 32
recreational substances, 61*t*
reflexes, 19
reflexive free thyroxine (T4) level, 21
regional patterns of atrophy, 50
relative contraindications, 49
REM sleep behavior disorder (RBD),
    97, 99–100
REM sleep without atonia (RSWA), 97
renal disorders, 213–14
repetition, 17–19
respect, 4
respiratory conditions, 130*t*
restless legs syndrome, 74
review of systems, 11
rheumatoid factor (RF), 22
risk factors
    for impaired decision-making
        capacity, 276*t*
    mild cognitive impairment
        (MCI), 73–74
    suicide, evaluation of, 186–88
    technology and, 288–89
rivastigmine, 81, 82*t*, 93, 98–99
Romberg's sign, 20
RPR (rapid plasma reagin), 21–22
RSWA (REM sleep without atonia), 97

safety planning, 190–92
salicylate levels, 21
SARS CoV-2 (COVID-19) virus and
    pandemic, 255, 285
schizophrenia, 241–46
Science Translational Medicine, 52–53
screening. *See also* cognitive screenings
    post-traumatic stress disorder
        (PTSD), 158–59
    suicide, 189
sedative–hypnotics, 61*t*, 261–62

selective serotonin reuptake inhibitors,
    111–12, 132–33, 140–41, 160
    for depression, 173–74
    drug safety consideration for, 168
    for OCD, 149–50
semantic PPA, 19, 104, 105*t*
sensory exam, 18*t*, 19
serotonergic medications, 61*t*, 140–41, 148
serotonin-norepinephrine reuptake
    inhibitors (SNRIs), 132–33, 140–
    41, 173–74
short-term memory, 72
single domain MCI, 73
single photon emission computed
    tomography (SPECT), 53–54, 97
6-Item Screen, 39*t*
sleep
    depression, 170–71
    over-the-counter sleep aids, 74
    tests for, 22
    VaD management with, 93
SLUMS (St. Louis University Mental Status
    Exam), 39*t*, 75
small-vessel disease, 91
SNRIs (serotonin-norepinephrine reuptake
    inhibitors), 132–33, 140–41, 173–74
social cognition, 62*t*
social dysfunction, 236–37
social history, 9–10
social isolation, 187, 188*t*
socialization, 81–83
Society of Nuclear Medicine and Molecular
    Imaging, 51
socioeconomic factors, 236–37
SPECT (single photon emission computed
    tomography), 53–54, 97
speech, 17–19, 18*t*, 26*t*, 28, 42*t*
SSRIs. *See* selective serotonin reuptake
    inhibitors
stability, mood, 29
standard uptake value ratios (SUVr), 52
stimulating medications, 205–7
St. Louis University Mental Status Exam
    (SLUMS), 39*t*, 75

stroke, 48–49
structural imaging, 46–50
subdural hematoma, 47
substance use disorders (SUDs), 142, 169,
    187, 188*t*, 257–65
Suicidal Ideation Scale, 171–72
suicide, 185–92
    delusional disorder, 236–37
    evaluation of risk, 186–88
    ideation with depression, 171–72
    OCD and, 148
    PTSD and, 158
    safety planning, 190–92
    screening, 189
    steps after identifying suicidality, 190
    thought content, 30
supportive care, 253
SUVr (standard uptake value ratios), 52
sympathetic nervous system, 136
symptomatic anxiety treatment, 131–33
symptoms
    psychosis, 220–21
    schizophrenia, 242–43
    of substance abuse, 261*t*
syphilis, 21–22

T1-weighted sequences, 47–48, 48*t*
T2-weighted sequences, 47–48, 48*t*
T4 (reflexive free thyroxine) level, 21
tamoxifen, 130
tangentiality, 29–30
tapering, 142
tau, 46–47
tau PET, 52–53
TBI (traumatic brain injury), 216
TCAs (tricyclic antidepressants), 168, 175
technology, 283–89
    apps and programs, 286–87
    assessing risk and
        troubleshooting, 288–89
    caregiver concerns, 289
    communication technologies, 285
    getting patients tech-ready, 284–85
    motivating successful use, 285

tools supported by artificial
        intelligence, 288
    wearable devices, 287
therapeutic activities, 81–83, 205
thought blocking, 29–30
thought content, 26*t*, 30, 235
thought process, 26*t*, 29–30
thyroid function tests, 214
thyroid stimulating hormone (TSH), 21
Timed-Up-and-Go (TUG) test, 118
tools, AI, 288
TPPA (*Treponema pallidum*), 21–22
trail making, 32–33
transcranial magnetic stimulation
        (TMS), 175
trauma, 59*t*, 159, 250
trauma-informed care, 288–89
traumatic brain injury (TBI), 216
TRD (treatment-resistant depression), 175
treatment
    agitation, 270–71
    Alzheimer's disease (AD), 80–86
    anxiety disorders and, 130
    apathy, 205–7
    dementia with Lewy bodies
        (DLB), 98–101
    depression, 172–75
    failure to thrive (FTT), 198–201
    frontotemporal dementia
        (FTD), 110–12
    mild cognitive impairment
        (MCI), 75–76
    normal pressure hydrocephalus
        (NPH), 120–21
    obsessive–compulsive disorder
        (OCD), 148–52
    panic disorder (PD), 136–38
    post-traumatic stress disorder
        (PTSD), 159–62
    psychosis, 224–26
    schizophrenia, 242–43
    substance use disorders
        (SUDs), 262–64
treatment-resistant depression (TRD), 175

Treponema pallidum (TPPA), 21–22
tricyclic antidepressants (TCAs), 168, 175
troubleshooting, technology, 288–89
TSH (thyroid stimulating hormone), 21
TUG (Timed-Up-and-Go) test, 118

undue influence, 280–81
uremia, 213–14
urinalysis, 21
urinary incontinence, 116–17
urinary tract infection, 120
urine drug screen (UDS), 21

vascular dementia (VaD), 59t, 89–94
    clinical insights for differential
        diagnosis, 66t
    pattern of atrophy, 50
    psychosis in, 222, 223t
Venereal Disease Research Laboratory
    (VDRL), 21–22

Veterans Affairs, 286
vision, 16–17, 30–31, 279t
visual hallucinations, 228
visuospatial and visuoconstructional
    skills, 42t
vitals exam, 16
vitamin deficiencies, 216
VP shunting, 120–21

wearable devices, 287
Wernicke–Korsakoff syndrome, 260
Wernicke's aphasia, 17–19
white matter disease, 50
Wilson's disease, 214
wisdom, 72
withdrawal, 22, 142, 216–17, 263
working memory, 42t

Yale–Brown Obsessive Compulsive Scale
    (Y-BOCS), 151–52